A CASEBOOK FOR
HEALTH CARE
ETHICS

Jay Ciaffa

Maria Kulp

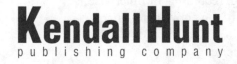
Kendall Hunt
publishing company

Cover image © Shutterstock, Inc.

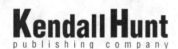

www.kendallhunt.com
Send all inquiries to:
4050 Westmark Drive
Dubuque, IA 52004-1840

ISBN 978-1-7924-9776-6

Published in the United States of America

Contents

CHAPTER 3   Reproductive Ethics   47

CHAPTER 4 Research and Technologies   75

CHAPTER 5 Behavioral and Mental Health   93

CHAPTER 6 Social Justice and Access to Health Care   107

CHAPTER 7 Public Health Ethics   129

Introduction

This text results from our several decades of collective experience teaching Health Care Ethics courses, as well as many years of service on clinical, educational, and public health ethics committees. We have always included case discussions in our courses, but in recent years our use of cases has become more extensive and intentional. Case discussions help students refine their understanding of key concepts and principles in the context of "real world" examples and provide them with opportunities to explore the nuances of ethical issues that arise in health care. More importantly, these discussions facilitate the development of skills and knowledge that will be most useful to students in their personal and, in some cases, professional lives. When students find themselves in ethically challenging medical scenarios, being familiar with relevant arguments and principles may be of some use, but they are more likely to benefit from the reasoning and communication skills that are developed in case discussions with their peers.

As we gravitated toward more extensive use of cases in our courses, we found ourselves yearning for a broader range of cases and for cases that facilitate critical and creative thinking by our students. Most medical ethics anthologies contain appendices of cases, and some of these have proved to be reliable teaching tools for us over the years. But, in our experience, many cases found in textbooks have proved less useful, due to a variety of shortcomings. These include: lack of relevant details or context, use of narratives that are inconsistent with medical facts or prevailing clinical practices, and lack of questions that encourage students to explore the broader implications of cases. In addition, many texts don't include cases on important topics that are of keen interest to our students, such as ethical challenges associated with public health and emerging medical technologies. To address these shortcomings, we gathered and revised cases from various sources, and started writing new cases based on our work in the classroom and on ethics committees. These efforts provided the impetus and material for this casebook.

Our aim is to provide a text that is adaptable to diverse courses and teaching methods. The text is appropriate for general education courses populated by students from various majors, as well as preprofessional courses designed for nursing and premedical students. In a course that focuses primarily on case discussion, it can serve as a primary text, lightly supplemented by topical readings and other resources. In a more traditional course, it can serve as a companion to an anthology of readings on key topics. Our cases include questions and suggested readings that are designed to facilitate in-class discussion, as well as further research and independent discussion by students. Our overriding concern is to provide cases that have real-world implications, and that will prepare students for decision-making in clinical contexts, as health care professionals, patients, and surrogates, and in broader social contexts, as citizens and civic leaders who contemplate policies pertaining to health care. Although most of our cases focus on clinical scenarios, we have avoided excessive use of technical language in order to promote accessibility to a general audience. We have included technical terminology only when it is relevant to ethical decision-making in a case, or when it serves an important educational purpose. For example, we have included details about medical interventions such as CPR and artificial nutrition and hydration, which are not well understood by the general public, and which are too often deployed as a result of default escalations of care.

The casebook is divided into 7 chapters, and readers can of course expect some overlap. For example, questions about professional roles and responsibilities are highlighted in chapter 1, but it should come as no surprise that they pervade most of the other chapters. We have included a Keyword Index to facilitate selection of cases and comparison of issues across different scenarios. Our lists of resources are intentionally minimal; they are intended to serve as a start but not a substitute for students who wish to do additional research on the issues raised by cases. References for cases indicate their origin.

The text contains 114 cases. Of these, four are taken almost verbatim from other sources and are marked accordingly as "From (original source)." Nineteen cases are substantially revised versions of cases from other sources, and these are marked "Adapted from (original source)." The remaining cases were written by us.

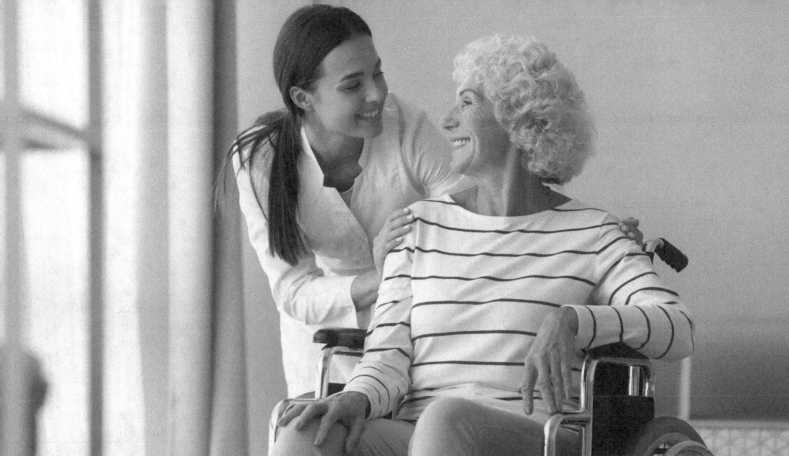

CHAPTER 1
Professional Roles and Responsibilities

1.1 Withholding Bad News from a Patient

Keywords: autonomy, paternalism, veracity

Dr. G is seeing a long-time patient, Lorenzo F, for an annual check-up. Lorenzo is 68 years old and recently retired. He is energetic and has had minimal health problems throughout his life, apart from intermittent anxiety, for which Dr. G has sometimes prescribed medication. Although Lorenzo smoked in his younger days, he quit cigarettes when he was 40, but still enjoys an occasional cigar.

Lorenzo tells Dr. G that he and his wife are leaving for a week-long "dream trip" to Italy in ten days. During the trip, they will meet several cousins for the first time, and they will visit the towns of their ancestors. Lorenzo mentions that he has had a nagging cough for the past few weeks, and he detected a small amount of blood after one coughing episode a few days earlier. He feels pretty good overall, but he wants to see whether he needs antibiotics before his trip, because he doesn't want his vacation to be ruined by an infection. Dr. G sees no obvious signs of infection, but he draws blood to rule out tuberculosis. Since Lorenzo smoked until age 40, Dr. G also schedules him for a chest X-ray the following week, "Just to be on the safe side."

Within two days, Lorenzo's tuberculosis test comes back negative, and Dr. G sends the result via voice message. A week later, the day before Lorenzo is scheduled to depart, Dr. G receives the radiology report, and the news is troubling. The X-ray shows a small but suspicious mass that is likely cancerous. Once the malignancy is confirmed by biopsy, Lorenzo will need to see a specialist for a course of treatment that will likely begin with surgery, possibly followed by chemotherapy, radiation, or immunotherapy.

Dr. G is conflicted about whether to tell Lorenzo this news prior to his vacation or wait until his return. He ordinarily communicates such results to patients as soon as possible, but he believes telling him now would likely trigger anxiety and could ruin his vacation. Also, a delay of eight days will not affect his course of treatment. For these reasons, Dr. G strongly suspects Lorenzo would appreciate getting the news after his vacation rather than before. Dr. G decides to deviate from his usual policy and delay disclosing the report.

Questions

1. Is Dr. G's decision to delay disclosing the radiological report justified? Does this decision infringe on Lorenzo's autonomy?
2. Does the long-term relationship between Dr. G and Lorenzo impact your reasoning about this case?
3. Should Dr. G have told Lorenzo that one purpose of the chest X-ray was to look for possible cancer? How much detail should physicians provide to patients about the purpose of the tests they order?
4. Under what circumstances, if any, do you think doctors are justified in withholding bad news from patients?
5. If Lorenzo lived in Italy, his doctor would almost surely wait to tell him the bad news. How does culture affect the ethical duties of doctors with respect to disclosing bad news?

Resources

AMA Council on Ethical and Judicial Affairs. "Opinions on Informing Patients." *AMA Journal of Ethics* 14, no. 7 (2012): 555–56. doi: 10.1001/virtualmentor.2012.14.7.coet1-1207.

Lagay, Faith. "Truth-Telling to the Patient." *AMA Journal of Ethics* (September 1999). Reprint of Antonella, Surbone. *Journal of the American Medical Association* 268, no. 13 (1992): 1661–62. doi: 10.1001/virtualmentor.1999.1.1.jdsc1-9909.

UW Medicine Department of Bioethics and Humanities. "Truth-Telling and Withholding Information." https://depts.washington.edu/bhdept/ethics-medicine/bioethics-topics/detail/82

1.2 A Depressed Patient Refuses Heart Surgery

Keywords: autonomy, capacity, depression, paternalism, refusal of care

John Q is a 62-year-old man with a wife and two grown children. He has just suffered his second heart attack in five years, and his cardiologist, Dr. Y, has told him that he must have bypass surgery, or he will likely die in the very near future. Dr. Y has also told him that because of existing damage to the heart muscles, John will experience some level of disability for the rest of his life even with the surgery. The prospect of being disabled is clearly distressing to John. He goes into a depressed state and refuses the surgery, saying he is "tired of being sick" and that life no longer has meaning for him. Despite pleas from his family, John is adamant about not having the surgery. Dr. Y and John's family believe that depression is clouding John's judgment and jeopardizing his life. They believe they should ignore John's decision and proceed with the surgery, as it is clearly in his best interest. They present the case to the Hospital's Ethics Committee for guidance.

Questions

1. Is John's autonomy diminished? If so, what factors are impeding autonomous decision-making?
2. Do you think Dr. Y does a good job helping John deliberate effectively about whether to have the surgery? If not, what would you have done differently?
3. Do you agree with the claim that surgery is in John's best interest?
4. Are the doctor and family justified in trying to persuade John to have the surgery? Are they justified in trying to force the surgery on John without his consent?

Resources

Kopelman, Loretta M. "On Distinguishing Justified from Unjustified Paternalism." *AMA Journal of Ethics* 6, no. 2 (2002): 75–77. doi: 10.1001/virtualmentor.2004.6.2.medu1-0402

Mappes, Thomas, David DeGrazia, and Jeffrey Brandt-Ballard. *Biomedical Ethics.* 7th edition, 41–45. New York: McGraw-Hill, 2011.

1.3 A Cancer Patient Prefers an Alternative Treatment Plan

Keywords: alternative medicine, autonomy, cancer, depression, refusal of care

Janet S is a 35-year-old woman who has just been diagnosed with cancer. Dr. B is explaining that the cancer has been detected early, which means that Janet has an excellent chance of a full recovery if she follows a treatment of surgery and chemotherapy. Janet is resistant, however, and says she does not want to have her body cut or poisoned by chemicals. She says she intends to follow an alternative treatment program, which includes a high-fiber diet, vitamin C tablets, and purified water. She expresses confidence that this will lead to her recovery. Dr. B tells Janet that this is absurd, and urges her to reconsider her decision, but she refuses. Noting that Janet has a history of treatment for depression, Dr. B suggests she should speak to a psychiatrist, but she refuses this suggestion as well. Dr. B concludes that there is no point in continuing to argue with Janet, and he wants to respect her right to make her own treatment decisions. He wishes Janet the best and tells her to set up an appointment if she wants to discuss the matter further.

Questions

1. Do you think Janet's autonomy is compromised?
2. Do you agree with Dr. B's claim that Janet's decision to pursue alternative treatment is not in her best interest?
3. Do you think Dr. B did his best to promote informed decision-making by Janet? If not, what would you have done differently?
4. When patients refuse interventions that appear to be beneficial, how should doctors respond?

Resource

Mappes, Thomas, David DeGrazia, and Jeffrey Brandt-Ballard. *Biomedical Ethics*. 7th edition, 41–45. New York: McGraw-Hill, 2011.

1.4 Parents Choose an Alternative Treatment

Keywords: alternative medicine, cancer, minors, parental authority, pediatrics, refusal of care

A two-and-a-half-year-old boy named Chad G has just been diagnosed with acute lymphoblastic leukemia (ALL). Dr. T informs Chad's parents that his overall prognosis is good, with the latest studies showing a five-year survival rate of more than 90 percent for children with ALL who are treated with chemotherapy. He also explains that Chad's chemotherapy will likely last for two to three years, with an initial phase of intense treatment followed by less-frequent maintenance treatments. Short-term side effects are likely, and include hair loss, nausea, risk of infection, and mouth sores. Long-term effects are less likely, but include learning delays, fine motor deficiencies, and heart problems. Despite these side effects, Dr. T expresses confidence that Chad will be able to lead a happy life with treatment.

Chad's parents, however, express grave concerns about chemotherapy, asserting that it will be too toxic and that it may not even help their child. They prefer to treat Chad's leukemia with a special diet of macrobiotic rice and Laetrile, an extract from apricot pits that is widely touted as a cancer treatment on alternative therapy websites. Chad's parents tell Dr. T that they have seen numerous uplifting success stories from cancer survivors on these websites, and they believe Chad will one day provide similar inspiration for other sick children.

Dr. T is deeply concerned by the parents' comments. He responds gently, saying he knows the information about Chad's diagnosis and possible treatment is a lot to process. But he wants them to know that there is no credible evidence supporting Laetrile as a cancer treatment, and that Chad's best and only chance for survival is chemotherapy. Chad's parents are clearly displeased with this rejoinder. They tell Dr. T that they resent being told what is best for their child, and they abruptly leave his office.

Questions

1. Should Dr. T follow up with Chad's parents? If so, how should he approach that conversation?
2. If Chad's parents persist in their refusal of chemotherapy, should Dr. T file an endangered child report with Child Protective Services? How, if at all, do you think CPS should intervene in this case?
3. When, if ever, should parental decisions regarding medical care for children be overruled?

Resource

Diekema, Douglas. "Parental Refusals of Recommended Medical Interventions." In *Clinical Ethics in Pediatrics: A Cased-based Textbook*, edited by Diekema, et al., 14–17. Cambridge: Cambridge University Press, 2011.

Reference

Adapted from Parks, Jennifer A. and Victoria Wilke. *Bioethics in a Changing World*. 1st edition, 788. New Jersey: Pearson, 2010.

1.5 A Mature Minor and her Mother Refuse Chemotherapy

Keywords: autonomy, cancer, minors, parental authority, refusal of care

Mary W, a 16-year-old girl, was recently diagnosed with Hodgkin's lymphoma. She had a lymphadenectomy to remove two lymph nodes, after which her mother, Jackie, checked her out of the hospital. Jackie and Mary explain to hospital staff that they wish to get a second opinion before continuing with treatment, though Mary's health care team urges Mary to start chemotherapy immediately.

When Mary's doctor, Dr. L, follows up with Mary and Jackie a few days after Mary was checked out of the hospital, Jackie explains that Mary does not want any chemotherapy. According to Jackie, Mary believes that chemotherapy would cause her great harm and destroy her chances of one day having children. Dr. L asks Jackie to bring Mary into his office so they can discuss this choice and Jackie agrees.

At the meeting, Dr. L explains that with chemotherapy, Mary has an 85 percent chance of survival. He does not deny that chemotherapy might affect Mary's fertility, but tells Mary that without chemotherapy, she is almost certain to die. Mary and Jackie listen, occasionally asking questions, but when Dr. L asks whether Mary will consent to treatment, she still says no. She says she understands she will likely die without it, but prefers death to poisoning herself and living through chemotherapy. Jackie tells Dr. L that she will support Mary's decision, despite knowing that it may lead to her daughter's death.

Dr. L is not willing to accept this decision. He believes Mary is being neglected by her mother, who has the authority to make her medical decisions, and he decides to seek a court order mandating treatment.

Questions

1. Should Mary and her mother be allowed to refuse chemotherapy?
2. Suppose Mary's mother sided with the doctor. Should treatment then be provided against Mary's wishes?
3. Suppose Mary wanted the treatment, but her mother refused to authorize. Should treatment then be provided against her mother's wishes?
4. Suppose Mary was 8 years old or 12 years old. Would these variations alter your assessment of the case?
5. Do you think the court should mandate treatment for Mary? When, if ever, should the courts mandate treatment for minors over the objections of parents?

Resources

Diekema, Douglas. "Parental Refusals of Recommended Medical Interventions." In *Clinical Ethics in Pediatrics: A Cased-based Textbook,* edited by Douglas Diekema, Mark R. Mercurio, and Mary B. Adam, 14–17. Cambridge: Cambridge University Press, 2011.

Goodlander, Emily C. and Jessica Wilen Berg, "Pediatric Decision-making: Adolescent Patients." In *Clinical Ethics in Pediatrics: A Cased-based Textbook*, edited by Douglas Diekema, Mark R. Mercurio, and Mary B. Adam, 7–13. Cambridge: Cambridge University Press, 2011.

Harris, Elizabeth A. "Connecticut Teenager with Cancer Loses Court Fight to Refuse Chemotherapy." *The New York Times*, January 9, 2015.

Relevant legal cases: Cassandra C. (Connecticut), Daniel Hauser (Minnesota), Phillip B (California).

1.6 A Doctor Refuses a Patient's Request to Modify Medication

Keywords: autonomy, paternalism, prescribing

Lila D is a professional ballerina who suffers from asthma, and she recently moved from New York to Chicago. Shortly after her arrival, Lila seeks out Dr. R, a highly respected specialist, to treat her asthma. In their first meeting, Dr. R indicates that he is proud of his track record treating asthma patients, and expresses confidence that he can effectively bring her symptoms under control. Lila is delighted to hear this. Dr. R prescribes multiple courses of steroids, which soon bring her wheezing under complete control. Unfortunately, Lila experiences some side effects, including minor muscle weakness and weight gain, which impede her ability to dance at a high level. She is distraught over her dancing and asks if Dr. R can reduce the dosage or try another medication. She points out that her previous doctor in New York was willing to adjust medications in order to accommodate her dancing. Dr. R responds politely but firmly that he is in the business of treating asthma, not accommodating the lifestyles, hobbies, or outside interests of his patients. He says other medications will be less effective, and he thinks it will be best for her in long term if she keeps her symptoms under control. If Lila wants to change or adjust her medication, she will need to find a new doctor.

Questions

1. Is Dr. R acting paternalistically in this case? Is his refusal to accommodate Lila's request an infringement on her autonomy?
2. Do you think Dr. R should accommodate Lila's request to modify her treatment?
3. Do you think doctors have a duty to accommodate the nonmedical interests of patients? What factors should they consider in deciding whether to make such accommodations?

Resources

Childress, James and Mark Siegler. "Metaphors and Models of Doctor-Patient Relationships: Their Implications for Autonomy." *Theoretical Medicine* 5 (1984): 17–30.

Modern Hippocratic Oath. https://www.pbs.org/wgbh/nova/doctors/oath_modern.html.

Reference

Adapted from Siegler, Mark. "Searching for Moral Certainty in Medicine: A Proposal for a New Model of the Doctor Patient Encounter." *Bulletin of the New York Academy of Medicine* 57, no. 1 (1981): 56–69. https://www.ncbi.nlm.nih.gov/pmc/articles/PMC1808387/pdf/bullnyacadmed00096-0058.pdf

1.7 Pressure to Prescribe

Keywords: parental authority, pediatrics, prescribing

Dr. P is a new associate of a small pediatrics practice that he joined immediately following residency. He feels fairly comfortable in his role, but is still getting used to the way the practice is operated. He is only given 15 minutes with each patient and often feels rushed.

Dr. P's next patient is a two-year-old boy, Johnny L, with fever and ear pain he's had for two days. After examining Johnny, Dr. P tells his mother, Linda, that Johnny very likely has a common viral infection that should resolve itself in a few days. He recommends children's Motrin for the pain and fever and tells Linda that Johnny should be kept away from other children until his fever has been gone for a day.

Linda is visibly annoyed. She asks whether an antibiotic can be prescribed, explaining she didn't skip work and make an appointment so she could be told to "wait it out." Dr. P explains that an antibiotic won't be of any help with a viral infection. He also explains that the overuse of antibiotics is leading to antibiotic-resistant strains of bacteria. He tells her that prescribing antibiotics unnecessarily could lead to Johnny and other children suffering in the future because they've developed infections that are resistant to antibiotics.

Angry, Linda snaps, "You're not the one up with Johnny at night when he's screaming and in pain. Just give me the drug. Your partner, Dr. S, would prescribe the antibiotic. He's given them to Johnny in the past when he's been sick. If this wasn't a last-minute appointment, I never would have seen you. I'm going to tell him about this when I see him next." Dr. P realizes that there is a very slight chance Johnny's ear infection is caused by a bacterial infection and that the antibiotics would present very little risk to Johnny if prescribed. He worries about what a complaint to one of the founding partners of the clinic would mean for his place at the practice. He wonders what to do.

Questions

1. Should Dr. P write the prescription for Johnny?
2. How, if at all, should the fact that Dr. P is new to the practice factor into his decision about what to do in this situation?
3. Are there policies or practices that could be instituted at the pediatrics practice to help providers more easily navigate this issue in the future? If so, what are they?
4. Providers are often required to balance the desires of an individual patient and the promotion of public health (e.g., when a parent refuses to vaccinate their child). How should a provider balance these competing obligations?

Resources

Allen, Thomas, Dorte Gyrd-Hansen, Søren Rud Kristensen, Anne Sophie Oxholm, Line Bjørnskov Pedersen, and Mario Pezzino. "Physicians under Pressure: Evidence from Antibiotics Prescribing in England." *Medical Decision Making* 42, no. 3 (2022): 303–12. https://doi.org/10.1177/0272989X211069931.

Jacobs, Andrew. "Doctors Heavily Overprescribed Antibiotics Early in the Pandemic." *The New York Times,* June 4, 2020.

Stivers, Tanya, and Stefan Timmermans. "Arriving at No: Patient Pressure to Prescribe Antibiotics and Physicians' Responses." *Social Science and Medicine* 290 (2021): 114007. https://doi.org/10.1016/j.socscimed.2021.114007.

1.8 Request for an Off-Label Prescription

Keywords: autonomy, paternalism, prescribing

Julie O is 18 years old and she just finished her first semester of college. Julie is enjoying college, and she has adjusted well socially, having made many new friends in campus, but she is struggling academically. Julie was a straight A student in high school, but she got Cs in three of her college classes, primarily due to low test scores. Her curriculum requires long hours of studying, and she has been prone to distraction, especially by the numerous social activities on and around campus. During exam sessions, she has trouble concentrating and remembering what she studied. When Julie discusses her struggles with friends, she discovers that several of them are taking medications like Ritalin, Provigil, and Adderall, which have really helped their academic performance. While some of these friends are prescribed the medications for conditions like ADHD, others have received prescriptions for "off-label" use—that is, to boost cognitive abilities, rather than to treat the conditions for which they were approved.

When Julie is at home on holiday break, she makes an appointment to see Dr. K, a family practitioner who has been treating her since she was a child. She explains her struggles and asks Dr. K whether he can prescribe medication to help her concentrate better in the upcoming semester. She is really worried about another subpar academic performance, since it could compromise her chance for graduate studies. Dr. K knows Julie well, and she has no history of ADHD, depression, or any of the disorders that are targeted by the drugs she is requesting. A brief examination confirms that she has not developed any such conditions during her brief time at college, which presents Dr. K with a dilemma. Dr. K knows that Ritalin, Provigil, and other drugs are commonly prescribed "off-label" for persons who are struggling with concentration in school or in the workplace. And he also knows that several studies and much anecdotal evidence suggest that the drugs improve memory and concentration in persons who do not suffer from neurologic disorders. But, unlike many of his colleagues, Dr. K is reluctant to write prescriptions for off-label use. The drugs were not intended for use in the normal population, and they have not been extensively tested in that demographic. He believes doctors should not be providing healthy patients with performance-enhancing drugs, particularly if there is any possibility of adverse side effects. At the same time, he wants to help Julie with a problem that is clearly affecting her college experience, and that could have long-term ramifications if it is not addressed.

Dr. K is torn and wonders what to do.

Questions

1. Do you think Dr. K should write the prescription for Julie?
2. If Dr. K refuses to offer the prescription, would his action be paternalistic? Would he be infringing on Julie's autonomy?
3. If you oppose writing the prescription, what advice do you think Dr. K should offer to help Julie address her academic struggles? If Julie continued to struggle after following this advice, would you reconsider offering the prescription?
4. If you oppose writing this prescription, suppose Julie is not a young college student, but a 60-year-old woman, whose performance in the workplace has been slipping due to normal, age-related diminishment of memory. Would you support writing the prescription then?
5. If you support writing this prescription, suppose Julie is a college soccer player, who asks Dr. K to prescribe a drug that might improve her athletic performance and that does not violate any rules. Or suppose she received Bs rather than Cs in her first semester. Would you support writing the prescription in these scenarios?

Resources

Larriviere, Dan. "'Doc, I Need a Smart Pill': Requests for Neurologic Enhancement." *AMA Journal of Ethics* 12, no. 11 (2010): 849–53. doi: 10.1001/virtualmentor.2010.12.11.ccas2-1011.

Mappes, Thomas, David DeGrazia, and Jeffrey Brandt-Ballard. *Biomedical Ethics.* 7th edition, 41–45, 48–51. New York: McGraw-Hill, 2011.

Reiner, Peter B. "Distinguishing between Restoration and Enhancement in Neuropharmacology." *AMA Journal of Ethics* 12, no. 11 (2010): 885–88. doi: 10.1001/virtualmentor.2010.12.11.msoc1-1011.

1.9 Accepting Gifts from Pharmaceutical Representatives

Keywords: conflict of interest, prescribing

Dr. N has a busy family medicine practice that he runs with two other family medicine doctors. The practice is 10 years old and since the beginning, one constant at the practice has been visits from pharmaceutical representatives. The representatives show up to talk with the doctors at the practice about the drugs their company manufactured, and they frequently provide samples of drugs for physicians to distribute to their patients. They also bring small gifts for the doctors and staff, such as flowers for the nursing staff, office supplies bearing the name of their company's latest drug, or lunch for the office. A few times, a representative offered Dr. N more expensive gifts—these included box seats to his favorite local baseball team's game; a dinner at one of the nicer restaurants in town; and an offer to pay for airfare, hotel, and registration fees at a conference on the use of new medications. Dr. N refused these offers, because he thought accepting these gifts crossed an ethical line in a way that accepting the smaller gifts did not. However, Dr. N is disturbed when he reads an editorial in a family practice journal that lays out strong evidence that accepting even these small gifts has a dramatic effect on a doctor's prescribing practices.

Questions

1. Should Dr. N continue to accept the small gifts from pharmaceutical representatives? Should he allow his staff to do so?

2. If Dr. N decides to prohibit gifts from pharmaceutical representatives to his staff, should he have a similar policy regarding medications samples?

3. Where should Dr. N draw the line between small gifts and gifts of larger value? Is it appropriate to accept an all-expenses paid trip to a conference that might have educational benefit for his clinical decisions or prescribing practices?

Resources

AMA Code of Medical Ethics. Opinion 9.6.2. "Gifts to Physicians from Industry." https://www.ama-assn.org/delivering-care/ethics/gifts-physicians-industry

AMA Council on Ethical and Judicial Affairs. "Code of Medical Ethics' Opinions on Physicians' Relationships with Drug Companies and Duty to Assist in Containing Drug Costs." *AMA Journal of Ethics* 16, no. 4 (2014): 261–64. doi: 10.1001/virtualmentor.2014.16.4.coet2-1404.

Brown, Steven R. "Physicians Should Refuse Pharmaceutical Industry Gifts." *American Family Physician Journal* 104, no. 4 (2021): 348–50. https://www.aafp.org/afp/2021/1000/p348.html

1.10 Investing in a New Imaging Center

Keywords: conflict of interest

Dr. M is an established orthopedist in a major city, who is part of a well-respected medical group. His colleagues see hundreds of patients a week, many of whom are referred for X-rays, MRIs, and other imaging. There are four imaging centers in town, all owned by the same medical corporation. Dr. M recently had a couple of patients who had difficulty getting scheduled for imaging in a timely manner, and his office assistant was treated rudely when she followed up. He wants his group to invest in their own imaging center, arguing that this will be more convenient for patients, and will offer significant financial rewards.

But one of his group partners, Dr. A, has serious ethical concerns about this venture. In his experience, despite the occasional "glitch," the imaging centers in town are more than adequate in terms of both quantity and quality. He also cites studies which show that doctors who invest in such facilities often start referring patients for imaging at a higher rate. He is concerned about the possibility of escalated referrals based on lax indications, and he worries that the group will create a conflict of interest between what is best for patients and what is best for their bottom line. He wonders whether this investment can be reconciled with the idea that the group's primary ethical responsibility is to their patients.

Dr. M responds by saying he is confident his colleagues will avoid unnecessary referrals, and an additional option for imaging will surely be more convenient for patients. He also argues that sending patients to their own imaging facility across town is no different from sending them to the small lab in their main office to have blood drawn and tested.

The partners ultimately side with Dr. M deciding that increased convenience for patients and lucrative financial rewards for the group outweigh Dr. A's ethical concerns.

Questions

1. Is Dr. A right to question whether this investment can be reconciled with the idea that the group's primary ethical responsibility is to their patients?
2. Does the financial incentive associated with this new venture create a conflict of interest?
3. What rules might the group adopt to avoid possible ethical problems that might arise with this new venture?
4. Is the availability of other imaging facilities ethically relevant to the decision about whether to open a new facility?
5. What legal limits should be placed on referrals that enrich the referring physicians?

Resources

AMA Code of Medical Ethics. Opinion 9.6.9. "Physician Self-Referral." https://www.ama-assn.org/delivering-care/ethics/physician-self-referral

Green, Ronald M. "Medical Joint-Venturing: An Ethical Perspective." *Hastings Center Report* 20, no. 4 (1990): 22–26.

Pellegrino, Edmund. "The Virtuous Physician and the Ethics of Medicine." In *Virtue and Medicine: Explorations in the Character of Medicine*, edited by Earl Shelp, 248–53. Dordrecht: D. Reidel, 1985.

Sullivan, Thomas. "DOJ Targets Doctors for Accepting Bribes in Exchange for Referrals." *Policy and Medicine.* May 5, 2018. https://www.policymed.com/2015/04/doj-targets-physicians-for-accepting-bribes-in-exchange-for-referrals.html

1.11 The Oncology Nurse and Informed Consent

Keywords: alternative medicine, cancer, consent, nursing

Michael E is a 46-year-old man with acute myeloid leukemia, for which he has been receiving chemotherapy. The treatment requires him to be admitted to the hospital and has significant side effects, including nausea and fatigue. Michael has received three cycles of chemotherapy, and he has two more cycles scheduled. Unfortunately, his disease has been progressing despite the treatment; he is worried that his time is limited, and he is tired of debilitating side effects. He wants to explore alternatives to his current treatment, and he mentions this to Nurse G, who has been with him for each of his hospital stays. Nurse G tells Michael that there are alternatives to chemotherapy, including stem cell transplants and holistic, natural treatments. Michael is surprised to hear about these options, which have not been mentioned by Dr. S, his oncologist. Prior to his next scheduled infusion, Michael does some research, and he decides to pursue holistic treatment at a natural healing center. He cancels his infusion appointment, telling Dr. S that he is thankful for the information provided by Nurse G.

Dr. S is angry when he learns of this. He charges Nurse G with unprofessional conduct, and he asks that her nursing license be revoked. Nurse G responds by saying that Michael has a right to know about treatment alternatives, and that Dr. S's failure to mention these options undermined Michael's ability to offer informed consent for the chemotherapy.

Questions

1. Was Nurse G justified in providing Michael with information about alternatives to his current treatment? If not, how do you think she should have responded to Michael's desire to explore alternatives to chemotherapy?

2. Do you agree with Nurse G that Michael's consent to the chemotherapy was not truly informed, because he was not aware of alternative treatments?

3. Should physicians have the final word in determining what information is presented to their patients?

4. How should nurses respond if they believe doctors have violated their patient's right to informed consent by failing to identify relevant treatment options, or by failing to present information that is relevant to treatments that have been selected?

Resources

American Nursing Association. "Code of Ethics for Nurses." https://www.ius.edu/nursing/handbooks/ pre-nursing-handbook/standards-of-performance/code-of-ethics.html

Kuhse, Helga. "Advocacy or Subservience for the Sake of Patients?" In *Caring: Nurses, Women and Ethics*, edited by Helga Kuhse, chap. 3. New Jersey: Wiley, 1997.

Reference

Adapted from Mappes, Thomas, David DeGrazia, and Jeffrey Brandt-Ballard. *Biomedical Ethics*. 7th edition, case 8, 711. New York: McGraw-Hill, 2011.

1.12 The Office Nurse and Informed Consent

Keywords: consent, nursing

Joan R is going through menopause. Her physician, Dr. W, wants her to begin estrogen therapy. After talking with the physician, Joan agrees to the therapy. She stops at the nurse's desk in Dr. W's office to pick up her prescription. In the course of their conversation, Nurse M realizes that Dr. W has not informed Joan that other options are available to her and there is wide disagreement about which option is preferable. Instead of taking only estrogen, Nurse M reasons, Joan could take estrogen together with progestin, or she could choose to take no hormones at all. Each of the options is thought to carry different potential benefits and risks.

Questions

1. Should Nurse M provide Joan with more complete information about her treatment options?
2. Should Nurse M suggest to Joan that she initiate additional discussion with Dr. W to obtain more information about her treatment options?
3. Should Nurse M express her concerns to Dr. W? If so, how should she approach him?

Resource

American Nursing Association. "Code of Ethics for Nurses." https://www.ius.edu/nursing/handbooks/
    pre-nursing-handbook/standards-of-performance/code-of-ethics.html

References

From Mappes, Thomas, David DeGrazia, and Jeffrey Brandt-Ballard. *Biomedical Ethics*. 7th edition, case 9,
    711. New York: McGraw-Hill 2011.

Used with permission of McGraw Hill LLC, from *Biomedical Ethics* 7/e, David DeGrazia, Thomas A.
    Mappes, Jeffrey Brand-Ballard, © 2011; permission conveyed through Copyright Clearance Center,
    Inc.

1.13 Informed Consent and Cultural Differences

Keywords: consent, cultural difference, paternalism, veracity

Akira M is a 70-year-old man who has recently moved from his native Japan to the United States with his wife, Yua, in order to be close to their son. Akira has been referred to Dr. R, a surgical oncologist, to discuss the results of an endoscopy and biopsy. Unfortunately, these procedures revealed a large cancerous tumor in his stomach. Akira and Yua speak very little English, so his son is present during the visit to assist in communication. After brief introduction, Yua takes Akira out of the room, allowing Dr. R to converse with their son. Dr. R explains the nature of the malignancy and that an operation is clearly indicated. Since the cancer is localized, the prognosis is good, with a five-year survival rate of about 70 percent. Dr. R tells the son that Akira must consent to the surgery and that this will require providing him information about his diagnosis, prognosis, and potential risks associated with the procedure, along with other relevant details.

The son resists this request, saying that his father will "wither up and die" if he is told of his cancer diagnosis. Dr. R responds by politely but firmly indicating she cannot perform the surgery without Akira's informed consent, to which the son responds: "You just don't understand 'the Japanese way'—in Japan, the word 'cancer' cannot be mentioned to the person who is ill." He asks Dr. R to respect their cultural practices, by allowing Akira to have surgery without giving him any additional details. Dr. R reiterates that she does not perform surgery on patients without their consent. She points out that there are many other surgeons in the area, and she suggests that they try to find one who will accommodate their wishes as soon as possible, because any delay could lead to a less favorable prognosis.

Questions

1. Do you agree with Dr. R's decision to not provide the surgery?

2. If you disagree with her decision, what additional steps, if any, do you think she should take before providing the surgery?

3. If you agree with her decision, how would you respond to the claim that she is jeopardizing the patient's health and not being sufficiently respectful of his cultural practices?

4. Should Dr. R attempt to communicate with Akira, with or without his son's permission? If so, how should she approach that conversation?

5. Would it be reasonable to assume that Akira has authorized his son to make his medical decisions? Suppose Akira has an advance directive that grants his son power of attorney for medical decisions. How would that affect your reasoning in this case?

6. Suppose Akira's son refused the surgery without discussing it with his father. What steps should Dr. R take in that scenario?

Resources

Gostin, Lawrence O. "Informed Consent, Cultural Sensitivity, and Respect for Persons." *Journal of the American Medical Association* 274, no. 10 (1995): 844. https://doi.org/10.1001/jama.1995.03530100084039.

Zahedi, Farzaneh. "The Challenge of Truth Telling across Cultures: A Case Study." *Journal of Medical Ethics and History of Medicine* 4 (2011): 11. https://www.ncbi.nlm.nih.gov/pmc/articles/PMC3713926/

Reference

Adapted from Veatch, Robert M., Amy M. Haddad, and Dan English. *Case Studies in Biomedical Ethics: Decision-making, Principles, and Cases*. 2nd edition, 138. New York: Oxford University Press, 2015.

1.14 Nurses Vote to Strike

Keywords: nursing

Nurse F is a nurse at a private, suburban hospital outside of a midsize city in the United States. She and her fellow nurses have been bargaining with the hospital for better wages and improved working conditions for several months. A key area of dispute is the hospital's mandatory overtime policy, which the nurses want to eliminate. This policy often requires nurses to work well over 40 hours a week, on top of dealing with over-filled units and a shortage of nurse assistants and other support staff. The hospital claims that the mandatory overtime is necessary due to a shortage of nurses, but the nurses claim the shortage is due to poor working conditions and pay. The nurses also argue that these working conditions have led to poorer patient outcomes. After months of tense and unfruitful negotiations, the nurses vote to go on strike. Nurse F wonders whether she should join the strike.

Questions

1. The nursing code of ethics states that the primary duty of nurses is to their patients, but it also emphasizes duties of self-care and duties to improve work environments. How should Nurse F weigh these various factors in her decision?
2. Should the ability of nurses to strike be limited by the fact that they are essential workers? If so, what limits should be imposed?
3. Besides going on strike, what other steps might the nurses take to improve workplace conditions?
4. More than a dozen states have laws that prohibit or limit the use of mandatory overtime for nurses. What kind of limits, if any, do you think should be enacted?
5. Federal regulations require Medicare-certified hospitals to provide adequate nursing staff to meet the needs of patients. How would you determine whether the hospital is in violation of this requirement?

Resources

American Nursing Association. "Code of Ethics for Nurses." https://www.ius.edu/nursing/handbooks/pre-nursing-handbook/standards-of-performance/code-of-ethics.html

Deering, Maura. "Understanding Mandatory Overtime for Nurses: Which States Enforce Mandatory Overtime?" *Nurse Journal*. January 20, 2022. https://nursejournal.org/resources/mandatory-overtime-for-nurses/

National Labor Relations Board. "The Right to Strike." https://www.nlrb.gov/strikes#:~:text=Section%208(g)%20prohibits%20a,Federal%20Mediation%20and%20Conciliation%20Service.

O'Brien, Roxanne. "Ethical Values and Moral Courage: Nurses in Collective Bargaining Activities." *Health Progress: Journal of the Catholic Health Association of the United States* 97, no. 1 (2016). https://www.chausa.org/publications/health-progress/article/january-february-2016/ethical-values-and-moral-courage-nurses-in-collective-bargaining-activities

1.15 Substandard Care by a Nursing Colleague

Keywords: negligence, nursing

Nurse R is a new RN starting her first job at Sunny Pines Nursing Home. Nurse R has always wanted to work with the elderly, and she is delighted with her new job. The facility is close to her apartment, the hours are favorable, and the compensation is excellent for an entry-level position.

Patients at Sunny Pines are largely bedridden and, subsequently, at high risk for a variety of skin conditions, which can lead to infections and other serious issues. Because of these dangers, newly admitted patients are carefully inspected for skin problems. They are given a head-to-toe assessment, with special attention to bony areas such as the sacrum, pelvis, elbow, and heels. The assessment is time-consuming and typically requires more than one nurse, since most patients cannot stand or even turn themselves in bed. The results are documented in the patient admission report, to allow for monitoring and follow-up care.

Skin care for the elderly was emphasized in her Nursing curriculum, and Nurse R recognizes the importance of the admissions assessment. Unfortunately, Nurse B does not seem to share this view. Nurse B has worked at Sunny Pines for 14 years and she is one of the senior members of the Nursing staff. But Nurse R has noticed that Nurse B never asks for help from another nurse when she assesses incoming patients, which makes Nurse R wonder whether she is conducting a proper skin assessment. Nurse R's suspicions are confirmed when she notices that several patients Nurse B has recently admitted have skin problems. When she checks Nurse B's admission reports for these patients, she sees no indication of skin issues.

Nurse R approaches Nurse B about these patients to express her concern, and gently suggests that Nurse B ask for help with skin assessments during admission. Nurse B responds by telling Nurse R to worry about her own patients. When Nurse R mentions this encounter to several other nurses, they nod knowingly and suggest she steer clear of Nurse B, who has been known to make life difficult for other staff members. Nurse R ponders how to proceed. She is deeply concerned about Nurse B's substandard and potentially dangerous care, but she does not want to create workplace tension. She considers speaking to the Nursing supervisor, but she believes the supervisor is a close friend of Nurse B, and she is worried she might jeopardize her position at Sunny Pines. Perhaps, it would be best to drop the matter and allow Nurse B's conduct to be assessed and addressed by more senior staff members.

Questions

1. What additional steps, if any, should Nurse R take to express her concerns about Nurse B's substandard care?
2. How should Nurse R balance her concerns about job security and workplace harmony against her concerns about patient welfare?
3. Is Nurse R obligated to ensure that Nurse B's patients are being adequately cared for?

Resources

American Nursing Association. "Code of Ethics for Nurses." https://www.ius.edu/nursing/handbooks/pre-nursing-handbook/standards-of-performance/code-of-ethics.html

Burman, Mary E. and Lynne M. Dunphy. "Reporting Colleague Misconduct in Advanced Practice Nursing." *Journal of Nursing Regulation* 1, no. 4 (2011): 26–31. https://doi.org/10.1016/S2155-8256(15)30314-8.

Greenlaw, Jane. "Reporting Incompetent Colleagues." *Nursing, Law and Ethics* 1, no. 2 (1980): 4. https://doi.org/10.1017/S0270663600000431.

Maurits, Erica E. M., Anke J. E. de Veer, Peter P. Groenewegen, and Anneke L. Francke. "Dealing with Professional Misconduct by Colleagues in Home Care: A Nationwide Survey among Nursing Staff." *BMC Nursing* 15 (2016): 59. https://doi.org/10.1186/s12912-016-0182-2.

Reference

Adapted from Veatch, Robert M., Amy M. Haddad, and Dan English. *Case Studies in Biomedical Ethics: Decision-making, Principles, and Cases*. 2nd edition, 159. New York: Oxford University Press, 2015.

1.16 An Inferior Heart Surgeon

Keywords: heart disease, nursing

William S is transported to an Emergency Room suffering from chest pain. He is diagnosed with a heart attack, and tests show significant arterial blockage. Dr. O recommends bypass surgery and would like to schedule the surgery for the following day. While William is discussing the surgery with his family, their friend Sally arrives. Sally is a nurse at the hospital, and she becomes visibly troubled when she hears that Dr. O is William's doctor. She suggests that the family should get a second opinion, because she believes other doctors are better at "maximizing positive outcomes." She is reluctant to provide additional information about her experience with Dr. O, but it is widely known among staff that Dr. O loses patients at a much higher rate than other local cardiac surgeons. A second opinion will require transfer to a hospital across town, but the family agrees. As William is being transferred, the nurse who has been caring for him tells the family that she thinks it's great he is seeking a second opinion, though she too is careful not to criticize Dr. O. The new cardiologist, Dr. Z, confirms the diagnosis, and agrees that bypass surgery is medically indicated, but he says they must wait at least a week before doing the surgery, in order to allow the heart muscle time to recover. William is discharged, and returns to the hospital 10 days later, where Dr. Z performs a successful bypass surgery.

Questions

1. Is it appropriate for Nurse Sally to recommend that her friends get a second opinion?
2. If Nurse Sally cares for other patients at the hospital who are under Dr. O's care, would she be justified in suggesting that they get second opinions as well?
3. What additional steps, if any, should Nurse Sally and other Nursing staff take if they believe Dr. O is not providing adequate medical care for his patients?
4. Should patients have access to information about the qualifications and success rates of surgeons?

Resource

American Nursing Association. "Code of Ethics for Nurses." https://www.ius.edu/nursing/handbooks/pre-nursing-handbook/standards-of-performance/code-of-ethics.html

1.17 Treating a Racist Patient

Keywords: difficult patient, nursing, race

Nurse Q is a nurse in the Neonatal Intensive Care Unit (NICU) at a small hospital in a midsized city. She has worked in the NICU at the hospital for 10 years and has gained the respect of the staff because of her competence and calm demeanor.

She enters the unit one day and sees a man standing next to an incubator. She introduces herself and asks to see the band they require all visitors to wear while on the unit. Without showing her his band or introducing himself, he asks to see her supervisor. She insists on seeing his band, and once he shows it to her, she leaves to find the charge nurse, Nurse R.

Nurse Q is disturbed by the man's behavior but pushes her concerns aside as she continues her work. About 15 minutes later, Nurse R approaches her and explains that she won't be caring for the man's baby. Nurse R, who is white, explained that when she walked into the room, the man rolled up his sleeves and showed her a swastika tattoo and told her that he didn't want any nurses of color caring for his child, especially Black nurses.

Nurse Q is upset. Although this is not the first time she's experienced racism in her job, this is the first time it has been so pronounced. She is not sure what to do and is further concerned when she sees a note on top of the infant's chart explaining that she isn't to be treated by nurses of color.

Questions

1. Should Nurse R have honored the wishes of the father of the infant?
2. Should Nurse Q do anything in response to being asked not to care for the infant?
3. Many people choose providers based on a provider's gender (for instance, some women feel more comfortable going to an OB/GYN who is a woman). Is this practice morally different from selecting a provider based on race? Why or why not?

Resources

Kim, Melina. "Patients Choosing Healthcare Provider Based on Race." *Voices in Bioethics* 6 (2020). https://journals.library.columbia.edu/index.php/bioethics/article/view/5903.

Waseem, Muhammad and Aaron J. Miller. "Patient Requests for a Male or Female Physician." *AMA Journal of Ethics* 10, no. 7 (2008): 429–33. https://doi.org/10.1001/virtualmentor.2008.10.7.ccas1-0807.

Reference

Adapted from Munson, Ronald and Ian Lague. *Intervention and Reflection: Basic Issues in Bioethics.* 10th edition, 836–37. Boston: Cengage, 2017.

1.18 A Difficult Dialysis Patient

Keywords: difficult patient, duty to treat, nonadherence

Thomas A is a 46-year-old man with end-stage renal disease. Thomas has been Dr. W's patient for several months, but during that time he has not adhered to the agreed upon health plan. Thomas consistently misses dialysis appointments, which results in him needing emergency dialysis. Thomas also has shown up to the clinic drunk and has verbally abused the staff as they try to treat him. Dr. W has spoken with Thomas about his behavior, and has warned him that she will have to dismiss him from her care and refer him to another nephrologist if he shows up drunk and belligerent again. When Thomas shows up to his next appointment smelling like alcohol and clearly intoxicated, Dr. W ponders how to proceed.

Questions

1. Should Dr. W refuse to offer Thomas dialysis at that appointment?
2. Assuming Dr. W allows for Thomas to receive dialysis at that appointment, should she follow through with referring Thomas to another nephrologist?
3. Under what circumstances is it ethical to terminate the doctor–patient relationship? How does verbal or physical abuse by patients factor into your thoughts on this?

Resources

Hashmi, Adnan and Alvin H Moss. "Treating Difficult or Disruptive Dialysis Patients: Practical Strategies Based on Ethical Principles." *Nature Clinical Practice Nephrology* 4, no. 9 (2008): 515–20. https://doi.org/10.1038/ncpneph0877.

Ripley, Elizabeth B.D. "Where Does the Nephrologist Stand with a Non-Compliant, Abusive Dialysis Patient?" *The Internet Journal of Nephrology* 5, no. 1 (2009). doi: 10.5580/187c.

Senderovitch, Helen. "The Ethical and Legal Dilemma in Terminating the Physician-Patient Relationship." *Health Law in Canada* 36, no. 4 (2016): 168–73.

1.19 A Belligerent Surrogate

Keywords: difficult family, disability, surrogate decision-making, violence against health care workers

Dr. F is a third-year oncology resident at a large urban hospital. His patient, Letitia T, is a 47-year-old woman who has experienced multiple hospitalizations with infection related to her breast cancer. Letitia is intellectually disabled and has been taken care of by her 45-year-old brother, Luke, since their parents died a number of years ago. Luke is unmarried and they have no other family, so Luke has made the decisions regarding Letitia's care because of her intellectual disability. Although Letitia is an "easy" patient, Luke is often angry and belligerent toward health care workers when he feels he's made to wait too long to speak to a doctor or if he feels he's being spoken down to. A month ago, when Letitia was in the hospital receiving chemotherapy, Luke pushed Dr. F. Security was called and Luke was removed from the hospital and told to wait in his car for Letitia to be done with her treatment. He was also told that if he ever touched a health care provider again, he would be barred from the hospital. Letitia was so upset at the altercation and Luke's absence that she almost couldn't be calmed down enough to finish her treatment. Dr. F, who has always gotten along well with Letitia, sat with her until she was calm.

Letitia's infection is not responding to the first round of antibiotic treatment, and Dr. F tells Luke that Letitia will likely be in the hospital for longer than was originally anticipated. Luke is incensed, and he screams at Dr. F. Dr. F considers calling security, but worries that if he does, Luke will be forbidden from accompanying Letitia to her appointments or visiting her when she's hospitalized. He worries about the impact on Letitia, who has no other family or friends to come to visit.

Questions

1. Should Dr. F call security?
2. How does Luke being Letitia's caretaker and surrogate decision maker impact your reasoning in this case?
3. Are there potential steps to be taken before barring Dr. F from the hospital that have not been considered? If so, what are they?

Resource

Gates, D. M. "The Epidemic of Violence against Healthcare Workers." *Occupational and Environmental Medicine* 61, no. 8 (2004): 649–50. https://doi.org/10.1136/oem.2004.014548.

1.20 Confidentiality and the Duty to Warn

Keywords: confidentiality, duty to warn, mental illness, negligence

Dr. X, a psychiatrist, has been treating 15-year-old Matthew M for attention-deficit/hyperactivity disorder and anxiety for a period of two years. One day, Matthew arrives at his therapy session very angry, because his parents have told him that he cannot go to a school dance since he is behind on his schoolwork. He tells the doctor that he feels his parents don't understand his situation and says that sometimes he "could just kill them." After some discussion, Matthew calms down, and the doctor asks if he was really serious about harming his parents. "Of course not," Matthew says, "You know I love my parents; I was just venting." Though some studies suggest a link between ADHD and violent behavior, Matthew has no history of violence or unstable behavior either at home or at school. Moreover, previous sessions have indicated that he seems to have a close, loving relationship with both of his parents, who are very supportive and attentive. Dr. X has worked hard to establish trust with his patient, and he fears that disclosing the threat could undermine this trust and his ability to effectively treat Matthew. Dr. X decides not to warn the parents about their son's threatening comment. Later that night, Matthew shoots both of his parents to death with a hunting rifle. Matthew's remaining family subsequently sues the therapist for failing to warn the parents about the threat.

Questions

1. Do you think Dr. X should have warned the parents about their son's threatening comment? If not, why? If yes, how do you think he should have approached this task?

2. What criteria should be used to determine whether a threatening comment should be disclosed?

3. When, if ever, do you think therapists should be held legally accountable for failing to disclose threatening comments when their patients subsequently harm third parties?

4. Do you think Judge Tobriner (author of the majority opinion in the Tarasoff case) would find Dr. X liable in this case?

5. Suppose Matthew had a history of violent behavior toward his parents. Do you think Judge Clark (author of the dissenting opinion in the Tarasoff case) would support warning the parents about the threat?

Resource

Tarasoff v Regents of the University of California. https://scocal.stanford.edu/opinion/tarasoff-v-regents-university-california-30278

1.21 Sharing Genetic Information with a Patient's Family

Keywords: confidentiality, genetic testing, privacy

Brandy V is a healthy 27 year old who visits a local clinic for a routine yearly exam. She meets with Dr. N, a physician who recently graduated from medical school and has been working at the clinic for a few months. Brandy's physical exam shows no problems, and Dr. N says that he wants to draw blood for some routine labs. Brandy agrees but asks if Dr. N can add some genetic tests to her blood work. She is especially interested in testing genetic markers that indicate the risk of breast cancer. Although she is estranged from her family, including three sisters, she believes that one of her maternal aunts died of breast cancer at a young age. This is the first time Dr. N has received such a request from a patient, but he has no objection, and a quick inquiry reveals that the clinic belongs to a network that covers genetic testing for actionable diseases, including breast cancer. He agrees to order the tests for Brandy.

Unfortunately, Brandy's test reveals a mutation of the BRCA-1 gene, which means her risk of developing breast cancer is about five to seven times higher than normal, and her risk of developing ovarian cancer is about forty times higher. Brandy is distraught but not entirely surprised, given what she knows about her family history. Dr. N advises Brandy of preventive lifestyle choices that can reduce her risk of developing breast and ovarian cancer, and he recommends regular screenings. He also tells Brandy that she should inform her sisters that she tested positive for the mutation, since they have a 50 percent chance of having the same mutation and, if they do, they will have a 50 percent chance of passing it along to their children.

Brandy strongly objects to this recommendation, telling Dr. N that she hasn't talked to her family since she left home at the age of 17 and she does not intend to do so now. Dr. N says he understands why Brandy would not want to talk to her family and he wants to respect her wishes. But he believes it is important for Brandy's family to get this information, so he requests her permission to contact them. Brandy rejects this request as well, saying they can get their own testing done if and when they want to learn about their genetic risk. She insists that no one should contact her family and pleads with Dr. N to respect her privacy and maintain confidentiality.

Dr. N wonders whether he should reach out to Brandy's family, despite her objections. He also wonders whether he should offer genetic testing to other patients in the future.

Questions

1. Should Dr. N reach out to Brandy's family despite her objections?
2. Do doctors have a duty to warn family members about propensities for genetic diseases that come to light through tests on their patients? If not, why? If so, what factors should doctors consider in deciding whether to disclose such information?
3. Are there potential negative consequences of disclosing information to family members?
4. If Dr. N continues offering genetic testing to his patients, what practices should he follow to promote the rights of patients and their families?

Resources

American College of Obstetricians and Gynecologists. "Committee Opinion No. 410: Ethical Issues in Genetic Testing." June 2008; reaffirmed 2020. https://www.acog.org/clinical/clinical-guidance/committee-opinion/articles/2008/06/ethical-issues-in-genetic-testing

Laberge, Ann-Marie and Wylie Burke. "Duty to Warn At-Risk Family Members of Genetic Disease. *AMA Journal of Ethics* 11, no. 9 (2009): 656–60. doi: 10.1001/virtualmentor.2009.11.9.ccas1-0909.

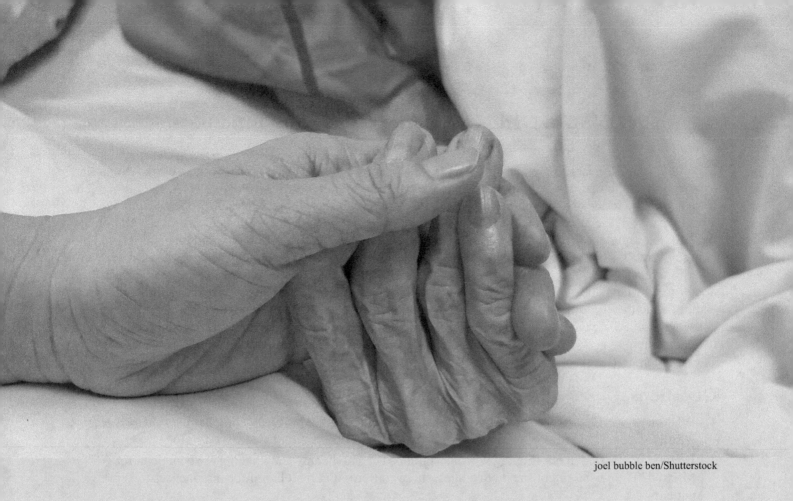

CHAPTER 2

Acute and End-of-Life Care

2.1 An Oncologist Orders Questionable Interventions

Keywords: cancer, consent, end-of-life discussions, nursing

Mildred P is an 82-year-old woman suffering from advanced bone cancer. Her prognosis is bleak, with a life expectancy of a few months at most. But upon the recommendation of her oncologist, Dr. A, she has agreed to an additional round of chemotherapy. The side effects are significant, and Mildred has been hospitalized as a result. Nurse T, the attending nurse, is concerned that the chemotherapy has little benefit and is compromising Mildred's quality of life, which is already quite limited. She believes Mildred would be better served by being referred for hospice care, where she would receive more focused and intensive treatment for her pain and discomfort. Nurse T is also worried that Mildred has only agreed to the treatment because she trusts her doctor to do what is best for her. When Dr. A orders a bone scan, Nurse T is further concerned that this procedure, which will require transport to an adjacent radiological facility, poses danger to Mildred, who is extremely frail. She voices her concern to Dr. A, who responds by saying that the imaging is needed to see if the chemotherapy is slowing the disease progression. When Mildred is being transferred, she suffers from a fractured femur. She is transferred to the ICU, where she dies 48 hours later.

Questions

1. What steps, if any, should Nurse T have taken to determine whether Mildred's consent to the chemotherapy is sufficiently informed?

2. Is Nurse T justified in questioning whether continued chemotherapy and imaging are beneficial for Mildred? If so, what might she do to address these concerns and limit harmful consequences to her patient?

3. What steps, if any, should Nurse T take after the fact, as a result of her belief that the oncologist ordered nonbeneficial and burdensome interventions, which ultimately harmed Mildred?

Resources

American Nursing Association. "Code of Ethics for Nurses." https://www.ius.edu/nursing/handbooks/pre-nursing-handbook/standards-of-performance/code-of-ethics.html

Kuhse, Helga. "Advocacy or Subservience for the Sake of Patients?" In *Caring: Nurses, Women and Ethics,* edited by Helga Kuhse, chap. 3. New Jersey: Wiley, 1997.

2.2 A Cognitively Impaired Patient Refuses Amputation

Keywords: capacity, consent, heart disease, refusal of care, surrogate decision making

Robert S is a 62-year-old man with a history of heart disease, and he has recently undergone quadruple bypass surgery. A month after the surgery, Robert returns to the hospital with a vascular graft infection (an infection in one of the bypass veins). Surgery is performed to remove the infected vein, but Robert suffers circulatory complications, leading to gangrene in his right leg. Amputation will be necessary to have any chance of saving Robert's life, but there is a significant chance that he will continue to have life-threatening conditions after the surgery, and there is a small chance he might not survive the surgery. Due to systemic infection, Robert's cognitive capacity is compromised—he is often unconscious or delirious, with only brief periods of lucidity. But during his periods of brief lucidity, Robert refuses to consent to the surgery, insisting that he does not want his leg amputated and saying he would rather "die whole" than undergo an amputation. A psychiatrist evaluates Robert and concludes he is not capable of making his own medical decisions. Robert's brother, who lives out of state, is the default legal proxy, and he asks the doctor to perform the surgery to save his brother's life. The doctor wants to remove the diseased limb, and he presents the case to the Hospital's Ethics Committee for guidance.

Questions

1. Would the doctors be justified in performing the surgery, based on concerns about the patient's decision-making capacity?
2. What weight should be given to the decision of Robert's legal proxy?
3. When, if ever, are physicians justified in providing medical interventions against the wishes of a patient?

Resource

Chow, Grant, Matthew Czarny, Mark Hughes, and Joseph Carrese. "CURVES: A Mnemonic for Determining Decision-making Capacity." *Chest* 137, no. 2 (2010): 421–27. doi: 10.1378/chest.09-1133

2.3 An Elderly Patient Requests CPR on Religious Grounds

Keywords: cardiopulmonary resuscitation, difficult family, end-of-life discussions, futility, heart disease, religion

Elise B is 78 years old, and she is hospitalized after suffering her second major heart attack. Tests reveal that her heart is severely damaged, and doctors conclude that she has very limited life expectancy. She has significant pain in her feet and toes due to decreased blood flow and she is also showing signs of kidney failure.

Dr. V, the attending physician, believes that hospice care is the best option for Elise, since it would allow her to be most comfortable in her remaining time. But Elise has different ideas. When Dr. V initiates a conversation about her bleak prognosis, Elise says that, as a Catholic, she believes "all life is sacred," and she asserts that her faith requires her to fight to the end. She wants to receive cardiopulmonary resuscitation (CPR) if her heart stops, and she wants to receive dialysis if her kidney function continues to decline. Her daughter Gail, who has been at the bedside through Elise's stay, supports her mother's decision.

Dr. V and his staff are concerned about these requests, as it is clear to them that Elise will not benefit from aggressive and burdensome interventions. Although Elise has decision-making capacity, she sometimes has trouble following what the doctor is saying, so Dr. V initiates a conversation with Gail. He explains that CPR is a burdensome intervention that will likely involve broken ribs for a patient as frail as her mother. Moreover, given Elise's age and condition, CPR is very unlikely to restore spontaneous circulation, and if circulation is restored there is a significant chance of neurological deficits if she regains consciousness. Dr. V wants to gently present this information to Elise. But Gail objects saying that this will only upset her mother and probably won't change her mind. Dr. V then confides that he is also Catholic, and he points out that Catholic medical ethics do not require interventions in circumstances where burdens are disproportionate to expected benefits. Gail responds angrily to this information, saying that her mother's religious beliefs are not his business, and that she strongly objects to him discussing the matter with her mother.

Despite Gail's objections, Dr. V wonders whether he should converse with Elise about the burdens associated with CPR, and about the requirements of her religious faith. He wants to respect Elise's wishes, but he believes he has a duty to be sure that her decision is sufficiently informed.

Questions

1. How should Dr. V respond to Gail's concerns about not wanting to upset her mother?
2. Should Dr. V converse with Elise about the burdens and benefits of CPR? If so, how should he approach this conversation?
3. Should Dr. V converse with Elise about the requirements of Catholic medical ethics? If so, how should he approach this conversation?
4. What other steps might Dr. V take to promote a care plan to best accords with the wishes and values of his patient?

Resource

O'Rourke, Kevin D. "The Catholic Tradition on Forgoing Life Support." *National Catholic Bioethics Quarterly* 5, no. 3 (2005): 537–53.

2.4 A Disagreement about Code Status

Keywords: cardiopulmonary resuscitation, code status, end-of-life discussions, heart disease, moral distress

Edna W is 88 years old and she is in the hospital following a mild heart attack. Though the damage appears to be minor, Edna suffered a major heart attack nearly 20 years earlier, after which she had quadruple bypass surgery. Since that time, Edna has also suffered two "mini-strokes," which thankfully have had no lingering effects. But the tests show that Edna's heartbeat is irregular, which greatly increases the risk of a major heart attack or stroke. The doctor explains that this can be addressed by inserting a pacemaker, which is a minor and relatively safe surgical procedure, but there are some risks, especially for an elderly, frail patient like Edna. The surgeon, Dr. M, tells Edna that there is a very small chance that her heart might stop during surgery, and he asks if she wants him to try to restart her heart with shocks if this should occur. She says "Of course, I'm having this surgery so I can go back to enjoying my grandkids!" The surgery is successful, but when she returns to the ward her condition worsens. Edna's heart rate is erratic and attempts to stabilize her are proving unsuccessful. Edna's adult daughters are at her bedside, waiting nervously to see whether her condition improves.

Nurse K has been caring for Edna throughout her stay and she is concerned about Edna's deterioration. She is also concerned that there has been no further discussion about whether to provide CPR if Edna goes into cardiac arrest. By default, Edna remains "full code," meaning that all resuscitative measures will be used if her heart stops. This is troubling to Nurse K, because she knows that outcomes of CPR are poor for elderly patients with advanced heart disease. Such patients are successfully resuscitated only about 10 percent of the time, and those who survive often suffer from broken ribs and cognitive deficits that require additional treatment. They are rarely restored to their previous level of functioning. She is concerned that Edna and her family have not been adequately informed about the benefits and burdens of CPR.

When she raises this concern with Dr. M, he says he has already talked to Edna about CPR prior to her surgery, and he is satisfied that full code status accords with her wishes. He sees no need to initiate a potentially upsetting discussion with Edna or her daughters while she is in such a precarious condition. Nurse K is upset by this response, and other members of the nursing staff agree. Excessive use of CPR is one of the most distressing aspects of their work—they are tired of watching patients expire after being "beat on" for no good reason, and they do not want to see this happen to Edna.

Questions

1. Do you agree with Dr. M that Edna's consent to CPR prior to surgery justifies her full code status? If not, what kind of follow-up is warranted?

2. If Dr. M does not yield, should Nurse K take further steps to address her concern about Edna's code status? If so, what options might she pursue?

3. Staff sometimes pursue a "slow code" or "show code" for patients like Edna, by "going slow" when patients go into cardiac arrest and by minimizing the use of aggressive measures like chest compressions and intubation, in order to reduce harms and allow the patient to pass peacefully. Do you think slow codes can be justified in such cases?

Resources

Forman, Edwin M. and Rosalind E. Ladd. "Why Not a Slow Code?" *AMA Journal of Ethics* 14, no. 10 (2012): 759–62. DOI: 10.1001/virtualmentor.2012.14.10.ecas1-1210

Semmens, Shana. "CPR: Advice on Helping Patients and Families Decide." *Elder Care: A Resource for Interprofessional Providers.* University of Arizona Center on Aging (2019). https://uofazcenteronaging.com/care-sheet/providers/cpr-advice-helping-patients-and-families-decide/

2.5 Access to Physician–Assisted Suicide for an ALS Patient

Keywords: neurodegenerative disorder, physician-assisted dying, rural health care, suicide

Roger B is a 67 year old who was diagnosed with ALS more than three years earlier. Unfortunately, his disease is progressing and symptoms have become more severe. These symptoms include loss of mobility, as well as speech and breathing difficulties. After considerable reflection, Roger decides he wants to make the use of his state's Death With Dignity Act (DWDA). Unfortunately, Roger lives in a rural town, more than 300 miles from the nearest major city in his state, and his local doctor does not participate in the DWDA because he believes dispensing lethal medication violates his fundamental duty as a physician. His doctor also expresses concerns about Roger's eligibility under state law. Specifically, he questions whether Roger meets the requirement of being within six months of death, noting that he has treated ALS patients who far outlived their prognosis. He also notes that once Roger is within the six-month window, his disease progression may prevent him from self-administering the medication, as required by state law, and he may also experience cognitive impairments, including dementia, which undermine the legitimacy of his consent. Though doctors in the nearest major city are willing to work with Roger to meet these requirements, working with these doctors will require multiple trips to fulfill waiting period requirements, and he will need an additional trip to fill his prescription, since his local pharmacy does not fill medications prescribed under the DWDA. Physician-assisted suicide is also legal in a neighboring state, and Roger learns that there are physicians who participate at a large medical center 60 miles from his home. But a phone call to one of these doctors reveals that they are only allowed to use the DWDA with residents of their own state.

Roger feels abandoned by his local doctor, and he is despondent and exhausted about the numerous hurdles he must clear to use the DWDA. But he is adamant in his desire to avoid the last stages of ALS. He wonders whether suicide by firearm is his only viable alternative, knowing he will need to do this while he can still load a gun and pull a trigger.

Questions

1. Is the doctor correct in his claim that physician-assisted suicide violates his fundamental duties as a physician? By failing to provide PAS, is he abandoning his patient?
2. What changes or exceptions might be made to the DWDA to allow patients like Roger to utilize the law? Are there potential dangers associated with making such changes?
3. In March of 2022, Oregon eliminated the state residency requirement in its DWDA. What is the rationale behind residency requirements? Should other states follow Oregon's example?

Resources

Craig, Alexander and Elizabeth Dzeng. "How Should Physicians Care for Dying Patients with Amyotrophic Lateral Sclerosis?" *AMA Journal of Ethics* 20, no. 8 (2018): E690–98. doi: 10.1001/amajethics.2018.690.

McMurray, Richard J., Oscar W. Clarke, John A. Barrasso, Dexanne B. Clohan, Charles H. Epps, Jr., John Glasson, Robert McQuillan, et al. "Decisions Near the End of Life." *Journal of the American Medical Association* 267, no. 16 (1992): 1229–33. doi:10.1001/jama.1992.03480160087040.

2.6 A Hospice Patient Seeks Humane Relief

Keywords: cancer, palliative care, physician-assisted dying

Dr. J recently moved to Oregon and has been working at Evergreen Hospice for three months. Her time at Evergreen has been rewarding, as she delivers compassionate care for dying patients and bonds with her coworkers in their shared mission. But Dr. J is now caring for a patient who has led to a difficult predicament. Harold P is suffering from throat cancer, and his symptoms are becoming more difficult to manage. Despite high doses of opiates, he experiences severe pain during most of his waking hours. He asks Dr. J to help him acquire a lethal prescription under the emergency provision of Oregon's Death With Dignity Act (DWDA). This provision would allow him to receive and use a lethal prescription within 48 hours. When Dr. J discusses this request with her coworkers, she is told that the hospice does not allow physician-assisted suicide. The director of Evergreen politely but firmly informs her that the mission of hospice is to provide comfort without hastening death. Dr. J responds by asserting that this is unfair to Harold. She points out that hospice physicians are allowed to use pain relief medications even in circumstances where these medications might hasten death. In light of this, she asks whether it is really wrong to help Harold access humane relief under the DWDA. When the director reiterates Evergreen's policy, Dr. J wonders whether she should increase Harold's pain relief medications to a level that is likely to suppress respiration.

Questions

1. Do you agree with the claim that physician-assisted suicide is inconsistent with the mission of hospice? If so, why? If not, when do you think hospices should accommodate patients who want to pursue physician-assisted suicide?

2. Is physician-assisted suicide morally different from use of pain medications that may hasten death? If so, how?

3. When hospices and health care facilities prohibit use of the DWDA, is this unfair to patients? Does this constitute a violation of patient autonomy?

4. Would Dr. J be justified in increasing her patient's medications to a level that is likely to suppress respiration? What other steps might Dr. J take to help her patient?

Resource

Cassell, Eric J. and Ben A. Rich. "Intractable End-of-Life Suffering and the Ethics of Palliative Sedation." *Pain Medicine* 11, no. 3 (2010): 435–38. https://doi.org/10.1111/j.1526-4637.2009.00786.x.

2.7 Euthanasia for Alcoholism

Keywords: addiction, physician-assisted dying

Phillip M is a 41-year-old Dutch citizen who struggles with alcoholism. As a result of his alcoholism, Phillip's marriage and relationship with his children have broken down and he was forced to move back to his parents two years before because he wasn't able to maintain steady employment. Phillip has been battling his disease for almost a decade now and has been in the hospital or rehab centers over twenty times during that period. Following another relapse, Phillip has managed to stay sober for four weeks. But he believes he will never be able to remain sober and worries about continuing to hurt his parents, as he is often belligerent and disrespectful toward them when he is drinking. After many years of uncontrolled and destructive alcoholism, Phillip concludes that his life is no longer worth living, so he decides to seek approval for euthanasia.

Although euthanasia is not legal in the Netherlands, it has been permissible since 2002. Acts of euthanasia are not prosecuted by the state when the patient's request for euthanasia is voluntary and well considered and when the patient's suffering is unbearable and intractable. The Netherlands has a medical organization, Support and Consultation on Euthanasia (SCEN), that reviews requests from those wishing to receive aid in dying.

Questions

1. Should SCEN approve Phillip's request?
2. Suppose Phillip's pain and suffering were due to an ailment that was not terminal but involved a lot of physical pain (e.g., multiple sclerosis). Would it be ethical to provide physician aid in dying? What if Phillip had a mental illness (e.g., schizophrenia)?
3. Are there relevant moral differences between providing physician aid in dying for a terminally ill patient and a patient without a terminal illness? Does the type of physician aid in dying (e.g., euthanasia vs. assisted suicide) matter?

Resources

Hewitt, Jeanette. "Why Are People with Mental Illness Excluded from the Rational Suicide Debate?" *International Journal of Law and Psychiatry* 36, no. 5–6 (2013): 358–65. https://doi.org/10.1016/j.ijlp. 2013.06.006.

Mendz, George L. and David W. Kissane. "Agency, Autonomy and Euthanasia." *Journal of Law, Medicine and Ethics* 48, no. 3 (2020): 555–64. https://doi.org/10.1177/1073110520958881.

Smith, Mark. "Euthanasia: One Family's Story." *The Times Magazine,* May 12, 2018. https://www.thetimes. co.uk/article/euthanasia-one-familys-story-3jl83tgbr.

2.8 A Patient Asks to Deactivate his LVAD

Keywords: heart disease, physician-assisted dying, suicide, withholding/withdrawing treatment

Marty B, a 62-year-old man, had a Left Ventricular Assist Device (LVAD) implanted for chronic end stage heart failure two years ago, hoping the device would help him to live until a heart became available to transplant. Unfortunately, Marty has experienced some complications since the LVAD was implanted via open-heart surgery. He has experienced chronic infections and dysrhythmia that have led to frequent hospitalizations. Even when he is not hospitalized, he experiences extreme fatigue, which leaves him unable to do much other than stay at home. Marty tells his cardiothoracic surgery team that he is tired of living in and out of the hospital and being unable to do the things that bring him joy, even when at home. He asks to have his LVAD turned off.

Dr. F, Marty's lead cardiologist, is troubled by this request. Deactivating the LVAD will almost certainly lead to his death within a few minutes to a few days. Also, despite the complications, he believes Marty is still a good candidate for a transplant, and there is a good chance that Marty will receive a transplant opportunity in the next few months.

Questions

1. How should Marty's health care team respond to his request? What steps should be taken to determine whether to accede to Marty's request?

2. In what circumstances should a patient be able to deactivate an LVAD?

3. How would you classify turning off the LVAD? Is there a case to be made that this is suicide or physician-assisted dying? Or is it better described as withdrawal of treatment? Is there a morally relevant difference?

Resources

Allen, Larry. "How Should Physicians Respond to Requests for LVAD Removal?" *AMA Journal of Ethics* 21, no. 5 (2019): E394–400. https://doi.org/10.1001/amajethics.2019.394.

Makdisi, Tony and George Makdisi. "Ethical Challenges and Terminal Deactivation of Left Ventricular Assist Device." *Annals of Translational Medicine* 5, no. 16 (2017): 331. https://doi.org/10.21037/atm.2017.04.39.

2.9 Removing Artificial Nutrition and Hydration

Keywords: advance directive, end-of-life discussions, heart disease, surrogate decision making, withholding/withdrawing treatment

Joseph P is a 79-year-old man who suffers from heart disease and diabetes. Although his diabetes is well-controlled, he has suffered two heart attacks in the last 10 years. He has an advance directive indicating that he does not want to be resuscitated if he goes into cardiac arrest. Joseph now suffers a stroke, which has left him paralyzed and semi-comatose. When he arrives at the hospital, a DNR order is written, but his family holds out hope that Joseph will improve. He is unable to swallow, so the family authorizes Artificial Nutrition and Hydration (ANH) via a Nasogastric (NG) tube. After two weeks and small improvement, the NG tube has to be removed, and it is replaced by a Percutaneous Endoscopic Gastronomy (PEG) tube, surgically inserted into his abdomen. Unfortunately, a few days after the PEG tube is inserted, Joseph suffers a second, much more significant stroke. Imagery shows a large region of his brain has been destroyed, and the prognosis is bleak. Joseph will never be able to leave the acute care facility or regain the ability to swallow. His life expectancy is probably short, but he could linger for many days or even weeks. When presented with this information, the family asks the attending physician to remove the tube, suggesting that their father would not want it under these circumstances, and citing the DNR as evidence. They are also concerned that artificial feeding will keep Joseph alive longer and in an undignified state. The physician balks at this request, arguing that the DNR order only applies to CPR, and indicating that he is not comfortable "starving his patient" by withdrawing nutrition and hydration.

Questions

1. Does Joseph's advance directive provide evidence that he would not want ANH in the current circumstances?
2. Under what circumstances should surrogate decision-makers be allowed to withdraw ANH? Do those circumstances apply to this case?
3. Is ANH different from other interventions, such as mechanical ventilation, which can also keep patients alive for extended periods of time in severely debilitated conditions?
4. Should ANH be morally and/or legally obligatory in cases where the patient's wishes are unclear? Should hospitals ever be allowed to continue ANH against the wishes of families in such cases?

Resources

AMA Council on Ethical and Judicial Affairs. "Opinion 2.20: Withholding or Withdrawing Life-Sustaining Medical Treatment." *AMA Journal of Ethics* 12, no. 12 (2013): 1038–49. https://journalofethics.ama-assn.org/article/ama-code-medical-ethics-opinions-care-end-life/2013-12

Relevant legal cases: Nancy Cruzan (Missouri), Terri Schiavo (Florida), Robert Wendland (California).

2.10 A Family Disagreement about Life-Sustaining Treatment

Keywords: advance directive, surrogate decision-making, withholding/withdrawing treatment

Shawn J is 32 years old and he suffered severe injuries in a motorcycle accident three years earlier. After being treated in the hospital for three months, he was transferred to St. Anthony's long-term care facility. Shawn requires ongoing medical support, and he will never be able to live on his own. One side of his body is paralyzed and he cannot walk or control his bladder and bowel functions. He is minimally conscious, but he cannot communicate or interact with others. He is being kept alive by a feeding tube inserted into his abdomen.

Shawn does not have a living will, and he never had discussions with friends or family members about his wishes in such circumstances. But his wife Megan insists that he would not want to be maintained in his current state. She notes that he was an outgoing person who valued his independence, and he once told her that he could not imagine going through life in a wheelchair. Since he was transferred to St. Anthony, he has pulled out his feeding tube several times, and Megan sees this as further evidence that Shawn does not want to live in his present circumstances. She asks his doctors to remove the feeding tube, arguing that state law gives her the power to make medical decisions for Shawn.

But Shawn's mother Sylvia vehemently disagrees with this request. Sylvia says she is not sure what her son would want, but she believes he deserves a chance to live. The care facility supports Sylvia in this disagreement. They tell Megan that their policy is to only remove a feeding tube when there is clear evidence of the patient's wishes, or when a patient is in the process of dying or in a permanent unconscious state. In all other cases, they continue tube feeding in accordance with their mission to respect life and protect the vulnerable.

Disappointed and angry, Megan resolves to pursue legal action.

Questions

1. Is the evidence presented by Megan sufficient to establish that Shawn would not want the feeding tube?
2. In cases of uncertainty regarding a patient's wishes, should family members have the authority to discontinue a life-sustaining intervention?
3. How should health care professionals respond if family members disagree about whether to continue a life-sustaining intervention?

Resources

Nelson, Lawrence J. "Persistent Indeterminate State: Reflections on the Wendland Case." *Issues in Ethics* 14, no. 1 (2003). https://www.scu.edu/mcae/publications/iie/v14n1/wendland.html

Relevant legal cases: Nancy Cruzan (Missouri), Terri Schiavo (Florida), Robert Wendland (California).

2.11 A Proxy Makes Questionable Decisions

Keywords: advance directive, capacity, heart disease, mental illness, moral distress, surrogate decision-making

Sara E, an 85-year-old woman, is admitted to the hospital in respiratory failure. She is placed on noninvasive ventilation, delivered via a face mask. Unfortunately, Sara does not improve. She has a history of heart disease and is showing signs of heart failure, and she is also receiving dialysis support. Though doctors believe dialysis support will be short-term, her prognosis is poor. Her life expectancy is very short, and she will not be able to survive outside an acute care environment. After 15 days in the ICU, the health care team recommends writing a DNR and transitioning Sara to comfort care. The only other alternative is to perform a "Trach and PEG" procedure, which surgically inserts a breathing tube in her trachea and a feeding tube in her abdomen. This procedure would allow Sara to be transferred to a long-term acute care facility for her remaining time.

Sara's oldest daughter, Debbie, has power of attorney (POA) for her health care decisions. Debbie does not accept the grim prognosis, and insists that everything be done to keep her mother alive, including the Trach and PEG procedure. She also asks for all of Sara's medical records to be forwarded to her primary care physician for a second opinion.

Sara has two other children, a son and a daughter, who live out of town. Dr. Z, the ICU pulmonologist, reaches out to them in a conference call. The son produces an advance directive written by his mother five years earlier, which he sends to Dr. Z. In this directive, Sara specifies that she does not want her life prolonged by "extraordinary" means, and she specifically identifies tube feeding and ventilation as examples. Sara's son also claims that Debbie, with whom he seldom speaks, has a history of paranoid schizophrenia. Sara's youngest daughter confirms this history of mental illness. Like her brother, she wants her mother's wishes to be respected, by discontinuing life-prolonging interventions, making her DNR, and transitioning to comfort care. But neither sibling wants to battle with Debbie over POA.

The care team is distressed by the use of burdensome interventions that are providing no benefit to Sara, and that appear to be contrary to Sara's wishes. But most believe they are bound, both legally and ethically, to follow Debbie's directives, since she has POA. Dr. Z is not so sure and asks for an Ethics consult.

Questions

1. What steps, if any, should be taken to try to reverse the decision that is being made by Debbie?
2. If Debbie persists in her request for all life-sustaining measures, should the hospital comply, or should they overrule and write a DNR order?
3. Would your assessment of this case change if the son could not produce a written advance directive, but still argued that his mother would not want life-sustaining interventions?
4. When, if ever, should health care professionals refuse to honor the decisions made by persons who have POA?

Resources

AMA Code of Medical Ethics. Opinion 2.1.2. "Decisions for Adult Patients Who Lack Capacity." https://www.ama-assn.org/delivering-care/ethics/decisions-adult-patients-who-lack-capacity

Traudt, Terri and Joan Liaschenko. "What Should Physicians Do When They Disagree, Clinically and Ethically, with a Surrogate's Wishes?" *AMA Journal of Ethics* 19, no. 6 (2017): 558–63. DOI: 10.1001/journalofethics.2017.19.6.ecas4-1706

2.12 Honoring a Living Will

Keywords: advance directive, cancer, capacity, consent

Esther K, a 65-year-old woman with a long history of diabetes, has been diagnosed with pancreatic cancer. At the time of diagnosis, she refused all aggressive therapies and she later wrote a living will stating that she did not want any "extraordinary means" used to prolong her life. She specified the "extraordinary means" as chemotherapy, CPR, and respirators. Three months after her diagnosis, Esther is admitted to the hospital in a confused state with discoloration in her foot and some evidence of necrotic tissue on top of her foot. Over the next few days, the necrosis spreads and she is diagnosed with gangrene. The surgeon, Dr. P, wants to remove Esther's foot to stop the spread of gangrene. Esther is somewhat confused, but she agrees to the surgery. Esther's family is very upset with Dr. P for suggesting the surgery and for considering her competent to give consent. They cite the living will as an evidence that Esther would not want the surgery, arguing that amputation falls into the category of "extraordinary means." They also argue that Esther is too confused to give valid consent, and they point out that she whispered to the nurse that she only agreed to the surgery because she was afraid Dr. P would no longer take care of her and order her out of the hospital.

Questions

1. Is this surgery consistent with the wishes expressed in the patient's living will?
2. Is the patient's consent to the surgery sufficiently voluntary and informed? If not, what steps should be taken to address this problem?
3. What weight should be given to the family's judgment in this case?

Resources

Lawrence, Ryan E. and Daniel J. Brauner. "Deciding for Others: Limitations of Advance Directives, Substituted Judgment, and Best Interest." *AMA Journal of Ethics* 11, no. 8 (2009): 571–81. doi: 10.1001/virtualmentor.2009.11.8.ccas1-0908.

Mappes, Thomas. "Some Reflections on Advance Directives." In *Biomedical Ethics*, 7th edition, edited by Thomas Mappes, David DeGrazia, and Jeffrey Brandt-Ballard, 363–73. New York: McGraw-Hill, 2011.

Reference

From Mappes, Thomas, David DeGrazia, and Jeffrey Brandt-Ballard. *Biomedical Ethics.* 7th edition, case 22, 717. New York: McGraw-Hill, 2011.

Used with permission of McGraw Hill LLC, from *Biomedical Ethics* 7/e, David DeGrazia, Thomas A. Mappes, Jeffrety Brand-Ballard, © 2011; permission conveyed through Copyright Clearance Center, Inc.

2.13 Following a Dementia Patient's Advance Directive

Keywords: advance directive, neurodegenerative disorder, withholding/withdrawing treatment

Albert H is a 77-year-old man who lives in a nursing home, suffering from advanced dementia. His wife died many years earlier, but he has an adult son and daughter, both of whom visit him regularly. Doctors and staff describe his condition as "severely but pleasantly demented." Albert is never upset or agitated, and he spends most of his time watching TV and smoking cigars. He enjoys talking to fellow residents and staff, typically telling them the same story repeatedly, as he quickly forgets what he has said. He no longer recognizes his son or daughter, but he enthusiastically converses with them when they visit, repeating stories that center on childhood memories. He appears to have no memories of his adult life.

When his dementia was first diagnosed in his mid-sixties, Albert executed an instructional directive in which he clearly stated that he would not want to receive life-sustaining interventions, including antibiotics, once his dementia progresses to the point where he can no longer recognize his loved ones. This advance directive was later supplemented by a POLST (Physician's Orders for Life-Sustaining Treatment) form, in which Albert indicated that medical interventions should be used only as needed for comfort. The problem is that Albert has now contracted pneumonia, which will likely prove fatal unless he is treated with antibiotics. Albert is unable to provide any input regarding his treatment, due to his dementia and the effects of the pneumonia. His children are aware of the advance directive and the POLST, but they believe the antibiotic should be provided, reasoning that their father's life, though severely restricted, seems to have value to him, and that Albert has no sense of the "indignity" he feared when he executed the advance directive. They believe treating the pneumonia is in Albert's best interests, and ask Albert's physicians to provide the antibiotics.

Questions

1. Should the doctor abide by the family's request to override Albert's advance directive? What factors should be considered in making this decision?
2. Would your assessment change if there was disagreement between the children about what to do?
3. Do you agree with the family's assessment that Albert's interests are best served by receiving treatment?
4. Is Albert currently the same person as who created the advance directive? If not, should the former person's wishes prevail over the apparent interests of the person who has pneumonia?
5. In general, when should the wishes of family members override the wishes of a patient as expressed in an advance directive or a POLST?

Resources

Lawrence, Ryan E. and Daniel J. Brauner. "Deciding for Others: Limitations of Advance Directives, Substituted Judgment, and Best Interest." *AMA Journal of Ethics* 11, no. 8 (2009): 571–81. doi: 10.1001/virtualmentor. 2009.11.8.ccas1-0908.

Mappes, Thomas. "Some Reflections on Advance Directives." In *Biomedical Ethics*, 7th edition, edited by Thomas Mappes, David DeGrazia, and Jeffrey Brandt-Ballard, 363–73. New York: McGraw-Hill, 2011.

Washington State Medical Association, Portable Orders for Life-sustaining Treatment (POLST). https://wsma.org/POLST.

Reference

Adapted from Mappes, Thomas. "Some Reflections on Advance Directives." In *Biomedical Ethics*, 7th edition, edited by Thomas Mappes, David DeGrazia, and Jeffrey Brandt-Ballard, 363–73. New York: McGraw-Hill, 2011.

2.14 Escalation of Care for a COVID-19 Patient

Keywords: advance directive, COVID-19, heart disease, prisoners

Darryl P is a 55-year-old man who has been transferred from prison to a local hospital for treatment of COVID-19. Darryl has many years left on his prison term and he has a number of health issues, including a history of heart disease. He executed an instructional directive several years earlier, indicating that he does not want life-sustaining medical interventions if he becomes gravely ill. Despite his symptoms, Darryl is able to communicate upon arrival, and he affirms the wishes that are expressed in his advance directive. But his symptoms worsen and, gasping for air, he agrees to the use of noninvasive ventilation via a face mask. Unfortunately, Darryl continues to decline, and doctors determine that he will require a transition to mechanical ventilation via tracheal tube in order to have any chance of survival. The patient now lacks capacity, so he cannot indicate whether he wants this escalation of care. Doctors are concerned that he is unlikely to survive even with mechanical ventilation, and they also worry that this escalation of care is contrary to the wishes expressed in the advance directive. The patient's only living relative, a sister living out of state, is uncomfortable providing input and says that she will support whatever decision is recommended by the health care team.

Questions

1. Should the doctors initiate mechanical ventilation for this patient? What arguments can be presented in support of treating versus not treating?
2. Does the fact that the patient is a prisoner create any special ethical challenges?
3. What weight should be given to the sister's input? If the sister insisted on mechanical ventilation, should the doctors abide by her request?

Resources

Lawrence, Ryan E. and Daniel J. Brauner. "Deciding for Others: Limitations of Advance Directives, Substituted Judgment, and Best Interest." *AMA Journal of Ethics* 11, no. 8 (2009): 571–81. doi: 10.1001/virtualmentor. 2009.11.8.ccas1-0908.

Mappes, Thomas. "Some Reflections on Advance Directives." In *Biomedical Ethics*, 7th edition, edited by Thomas Mappes, David DeGrazia, and Jeffrey Brandt-Ballard, 363–73. New York: McGraw-Hill, 2011.

2.15 Treatment Decisions for an Unrepresented Patient

Keywords: bias, cancer, homelessness, surrogate decision-making, withholding/withdrawing treatment

Dr. M is a new physician, working at a major urban hospital, and she soon encounters a familiar problem among ICU physicians. The city has a large population of homeless persons, many of whom show up for treatment at the ER for ongoing medical conditions. When she begins her shift, Dr. M assesses Trent D, a 79-year-old homeless man who was transported to the ER two days ago with signs of acute kidney failure, including severe swelling in his limbs and shortness of breath. Trent was stabilized through dialysis, but he is unable to participate in his care decisions, due to confusion associated with dementia, a condition noted in previous trips to the ER. Dr. M orders a CT scan, which reveals numerous tumors in Trent's brain. The tumors are subsequently determined to be metastases from previously undiagnosed melanoma. A consultation with oncology indicates that Trent is not a viable candidate for immunotherapy or other curative measures. Trent's mental capacity is worsening, and he is unable to understand his condition or his treatment options. Unfortunately, he has no advance directive that might provide a clue to his preferences, and a note in his chart from a previous ER visit states that he has no living family members. The hospital is unable to identify any friends or acquaintances who might help with his medical decisions.

After Trent has been in the ICU for two weeks, Dr. M meets with other members of the care team to discuss his care plan. The key question is whether he should continue to receive dialysis. Without dialysis, he will likely survive for no more than two weeks. With dialysis, he could live for 12 weeks or perhaps longer, before succumbing to cancer. If dialysis is stopped, Trent can be transferred to a nearby hospice facility, where he will receive expert palliative care in his remaining days. Continued dialysis may be possible at a skilled nursing facility, but it will be a challenge to find a facility that is willing and able to take a patient in this condition. Unless transfer can be arranged, continued dialysis would need to be administered at the hospital.

Dr. T, an experienced hospitalist, notes that the decision to stop dialysis "technically" requires guardianship proceedings in their state. But he quickly points out that physicians do not always "go by the book" in such cases, particularly when it seems clear that a particular decision is in the best interests of the patient. He explains that the court process is slow and there is a shortage of guardians in the state, which means that Trent could be dead from cancer by the time a guardian is appointed and acts. More important, he says, pursuing guardianship will do little more than extend Trent's suffering. For a patient of Trent's age with untreatable metastatic cancer, dialysis would be provided if requested by the patient or his surrogate, but it is not recommended by clinicians and is often declined by patients. "Why prolong this guy's agony? He has no family, so there's zero chance of a lawsuit. Let's do this right thing and transfer him to hospice."

Like other members of the healthcare team, Dr. M is inclined to agree that transfer to hospice is in Trent's best interest. But she worries about the implications of physicians making such a decision without any oversight. In her brief time on the job, she has seen evidence of homeless patients being viewed by staff as "socially undesirable" and a drain on resources. She wonders whether a current shortage of beds at the hospital is playing a role in Dr. T's assessment of what is "best for Trent."

Questions

1. Do you agree with the decision to discontinue dialysis and transfer Trent to hospice?
2. Who should make decisions regarding the cessation of life-sustaining interventions for unrepresented patients? What criteria and procedures should guide these decisions?
3. What are the most significant ethical challenges associated with treatment decisions for unrepresented patients in acute care settings? How might these challenges be addressed?

Resources

Chaet, Danielle Hahn. "AMA Code of Medical Ethics' Opinions Related to Unrepresented Patients." *AMA Journal of Ethics* 21, no. 7 (2019): E600–02. doi: 10.1001/amajethics.2019.600

Hulkower, Adira, Sarah Garijo-Garde, and Lauren S. Flicker. "Should Dialysis Be Stopped for an Unrepresented Patient with Metastatic Cancer?" *AMA Journal of Ethics* 21, no. 7 (2019): E575–81. doi: 10.1001/amajethics.2019.575.

Pope, Thaddeus. "Five Things Clinicians Should Know When Caring for Unrepresented Patients." *AMA Journal of Ethics* 21, no. 7 (2019): E582–86. doi: 10.1001/amajethics.2019.582.

Schweikart, Scott J. "Who Makes Decisions for Incapacitated Patients Who Have No Surrogate or Advance Directive?" *AMA Journal of Ethics* 21, no. 7 (2019): E587–93. doi: 10.1001/amajethics.2019.587.

2.16 Aggressive Interventions for a Patient in a Persistent Vegetative State

Keywords: end-of-life discussions, futility, persistent vegetative state, surrogate decision-making, withholding/withdrawing treatment

Mike P, a 38-year-old man, was involved in a catastrophic bicycle accident that sent him to City Hospital's trauma center. Testing revealed that Mike had suffered a traumatic brain injury and he was transferred to the ICU for observation four weeks ago. Since his accident, Mike has not regained consciousness and has remained in a persistent vegetative state. He requires mechanical ventilation to continue breathing. Despite aggressive care, further testing has indicated that Mike will likely never recover consciousness and that his brain injury will very likely lead to his death within a few weeks or months, depending on the aggressiveness of care administered. Dr. K, the lead doctor on Mike's care team at the hospital, suggests to his wife, Betty, that she should consider removing Mike from ventilation and to a floor where he would only receive comfort care. Failing that, she asks her to sign a do not resuscitate order. Betty refuses and is incensed that the doctor would even make these suggestions. She insists that all aggressive measures be continued.

Questions

1. If you were in Dr. K's position, what would you do in this situation? What are Dr. K's professional obligations in this case?

2. Assume you are an ethicist brought in to offer a consultation. How would you handle the situation? What conversations might you have?

3. If the patient's wife continues to insist that all doctors "do everything," would doctors be justified in withholding CPR or other aggressive interventions on grounds of "futility"?

Resources

UW Medicine Department of Bioethics and Humanities. "Futility." Accessed September 15, 2022. https://depts.washington.edu/bhdept/ethics-medicine/bioethics-topics/detail/65.

Welie, Jos V.M. and Henk AMJ ten Have. "The Ethics of Forgoing Life-Sustaining Treatment: Theoretical Considerations and Clinical Decision Making." *Multidisciplinary Respiratory Medicine* 9, no. 1 (2014): 14. https://doi.org/10.1186/2049-6958-9-14.

Wilkinson, Dominic J.C. and Julian Savulescu. "Knowing When to Stop: Futility in the ICU." *Current Opinion in Anaesthesiology* 24, no. 2 (2011): 160–65. https://doi.org/10.1097/ACO.0b013e328343c5af.

2.17 A Patient Resists Hospice Care

Keywords: end-of-life discussions, futility, palliative care, resource allocation

Samuel P, a 34-year-old patient, has been in the hospital for more than six weeks for treatment of a large, infected wound in his lower spine. Samuel suffers from spina bifida and multiple comorbidities, including kidney disease, for which he requires dialysis. His wound has not been responsive to repeated rounds of powerful antibiotics, and due to the location and extent of the wound it cannot be treated surgically. The treating physicians have determined that his wound is very unlikely to heal. The lead physician, Dr. W, informs Samuel of his grim prognosis, and tells him that no viable interventions are available to allow his wound to heal. She tells Samuel that they need to transition him from IV to oral pain meds so he can be discharged from the hospital. She recommends transfer to an inpatient hospice facility, which will be able to provide more extensive and beneficial palliative care as opposed to home hospice. In addition to being concerned about what is best for Samuel, Dr. W is also concerned that Samuel is taking up a valuable ICU bed: the hospital is near capacity due to an influx of COVID-19 patients, and it is having to turn away patients with a variety of conditions, including treatable cancers.

Samuel is conscious and has decision-making capacity, and he tells Dr. W that he is not ready to transition to comfort-only care. He wants to receive additional rounds of antibiotics and stay on IV pain medications; he is holding out hope that he will respond to a different kind of antibiotic, and he tells the doctor that oral meds do not effectively control his pain. If the hospital can longer care for him, he asks to be transferred to a rehab facility for further treatment. Dr. W responds by saying that no rehab facility will take him, since they would not have clear and viable goals of care. Also, a rehab facility cannot administer IV pain meds. Samuel could be discharged to his home, but his elderly mother and his sister, with whom he lives, worry about their ability to care for him.

Dr. W is perplexed by her inability to guide Samuel toward the most effective treatment option, and she wonders what to do next. She could give him one more round of antibiotics, which would allow him time to process his situation and perhaps convince him that the wound will not heal. Or she could start weaning him from IV meds, in order to prepare Samuel for discharge and perhaps convince him of the need for hospice. She asks for a consultation from the Hospital Ethics Committee.

Questions

1. Should Dr. W provide another round of antibiotics, despite agreement by the care team that it is very unlikely to cure the infection? Would this amount to administering a futile intervention?

2. Should Dr. W insist on discharge and start transitioning Samuel to oral pain medications, even if these medications will not be as effective? Could this be interpreted as coercing Samuel toward hospice care by increasing his pain?

3. Do you agree with Dr. W that entering a hospice facility is the best choice for Samuel? If not, why? If so, what might be done to help Samuel appreciate the benefits of hospice?

4. Does scarcity of ICU beds justify moving Samuel toward discharge as quickly as possible?

5. If Samuel insists on going home, what steps might be taken to help him prepare for this transition? Is the hospital responsible for helping Samuel and his family prepare for the challenges associated with home care?

Resources

AMA, Council on Ethical and Judicial Affairs. "Medical Futility in End-of-Life Care." *Journal of the American Medical Association* 281, no. 10 (1999): 937–41.

Dolgin, Janet L., Erin Sarzynski, and Wayne Shelton. "When Is Hospital Discharge Unsafe?" Relias Media Medical Ethics Advisor. May 1, 2016. https://www.reliasmedia.com/articles/137775-is-hospital-discharge-unsafe-ethical-response-is-needed

2.18 Aggressive Interventions for a Severely Impaired Neonate

Keywords: impaired infants, parental authority, pediatrics, religion, surrogate decision-making

Baby A is born with multiple impairments, including spina bifida (an opening in the spinal column), hydrocephalus (fluid on the brain), and microcephaly (a small brain and head). She also has a serious heart defect. Doctors at St. Francis Hospital tell her parents that Baby A will only have a chance to survive if she undergoes surgeries to close the opening on her spine, drain the fluid from her brain, and repair the defect in her heart. These surgeries will be painful and there is no guarantee that they will be successful. If Baby A survives, she may be able to go home after an extended stay in the Neonatal ICU. But doctors emphasize that Baby A will have a limited life expectancy and major limitations even with the surgeries. She can perhaps live to age 20, but she will likely be paralyzed, have epilepsy, and have severe brain damage, among other potential health issues. She will not be able to interact meaningfully with her environment or create relationships with others. She will require continued medical attention, including additional surgeries, and her medical conditions will be a source of ongoing pain and discomfort.

In light of this grim prognosis, Baby A's doctors suggest less aggressive treatment, including the administration of nutrition and use of antibiotics and bandages as needed. They recommend forgoing surgeries, in favor of palliative measures that will focus on making Baby A as comfortable as possible.

Baby A's parents, however, are horrified at the suggestion that not everything possible be done for their daughter. They insist on the surgery and any other treatments that will prolong their daughter's life. They also express surprise that doctors at a Catholic hospital, which is supposed to emphasize the sanctity of life, would suggest such a course of action.

Questions

1. Do you agree with the medical team's recommendation that Baby A be transitioned to comfort care? If not, why? If so, how do you think the medical team should respond to the family's rejection of this recommendation?

2. Would withholding interventions from Baby A contradict the idea that her life has inherent value and dignity? Do Catholic ethical principles require using medical interventions to extend life whenever possible?

3. Should medical professionals always defer to parents who want life-sustaining interventions for their children? If not, when should doctors be able to overrule a parent's request for interventions?

Resources

Aviv, Rachel. "What Does It Mean to Die?" *The New Yorker,* January 29, 2018. https://www.newyorker.com/magazine/2018/02/05/what-does-it-mean-to-die.

Caplan, Arthur and Cynthia B. Cohen. "Imperiled Newborns." *Hastings Center Report* 17, no. 6 (1987): 5. https://doi.org/10.2307/3563441.

Friedrich, Annie B., and Jason T. Eberl. "Catholic Perspective on Decision-Making for Critically Ill Newborns and Infants." *Children* 9, no. 2 (2022): 207. https://doi.org/10.3390/children9020207

Glover, Jacqueline J. and Cindy Hylton Rushton. "From Baby Doe to Baby K: Evolving Challenges in Pediatric Ethics." *Journal of Law, Medicine and Ethics* 23, no. 1 (1995): 5–6. https://doi.org/10.1111/j.1748-720X.1995.tb01322.x.

White, Michael. "The End at the Beginning." *The Ochsner Journal* 11, no. 4 (2011): 309–16. https://www.ncbi.nlm.nih.gov/pmc/articles/PMC3241062/

Relevant legal cases: Charlie Gard (UK), Baby K (Virginia), Tinsley Lewis (Texas), Jahi McMath (California).

2.19 Withholding Life-Sustaining Surgery from a Neonate with Down Syndrome

Keywords: disability, impaired infants, moral distress, parental authority, pediatrics, withholding/withdrawing treatment

Baby D is born with Down Syndrome (trisomy 21), a disease characterized by physical abnormalities, including a flattened face and upwardly slanting eye lids, and mild to moderate cognitive impairments. She also has a blockage in her esophagus, which prevents passage of food. The blockage is easily fixed through a surgery that has few risks and is almost always successful.

Dr. O, the family obstetrician, tells the parents that there are worse birth defects than Down Syndrome, but he wants them to know that Baby D will never live a normal life. She will require special education and medical care, and she will almost certainly never be able to live on her own. Dr. O also points out that persons with Down Syndrome are at increased risk for leukemia, immune disorders and, especially, dementia. After a brief discussion, the parents decide not to authorize the surgery. They tell Dr. O that they have limited financial means and they only want one child. They don't think they can manage the special care that Baby D will require, especially in her adult years. The couple is well into their 30s and the husband, the primary breadwinner, has significant health problems of his own. They wonder what will happen to Baby D when they die, especially if she develops major health issues.

Dr. O conveys the parent's decision to the Neonatal ICU staff, indicating that tube feeding should be discontinued, and Baby D should be transitioned to comfort-only care. This causes significant distress among ICU staff, who believe Baby D is being discriminated against and marked for death because of a relatively mild impairment. They ask the Ethics Committee to review the case, and they ask whether the hospital's legal counsel can pursue a court order to mandate treatment for Baby D.

Questions

1. Are the parents ethically justified in refusing to authorize treatment in these circumstances?
2. If you agree that treatment is morally obligatory, what steps might the hospital take to reverse the parent's decision?
3. Should treatment for imperiled neonates be mandated by federal law, state law, or institutional policies? If not, why? If so, when should treatment be mandatory?

Resources

Annas, George J. "The Case of Baby Jane Doe: Child Abuse or Unlawful Federal Intervention?" *American Journal of Public Health* 74, no. 7 (1984): 727–29. https://ajph.aphapublications.org/doi/pdf/10.2105/AJPH.74.7.727.

Resnik, Jack, "The Baby Doe Rules (1984)." *Embryo Project Encyclopedia*. May 12, 2011. http://embryo.asu.edu/handle/10776/2103.

White, Michael. "The End at the Beginning." *The Ochsner Journal* 11, no. 4 (2011): 309–16. https://www.ncbi.nlm.nih.gov/pmc/articles/PMC3241062/

2.20 A Disagreement over Resuscitating a Premature Infant

Keywords: impaired infants, parental authority, pediatrics, withholding/withdrawing treatment

Melanie M is admitted to the hospital showing signs of premature labor. An ultrasound shows that her fetus weighs approximately 568 grams (about 1.25 pounds) and has a gestational age of about 23 weeks, approximately 14 weeks short of full-term. Melanie and her husband are informed by the attending obstetrician, Dr. L, that data are not promising for infants that are born so early. Only about a third survive to discharge, and of those at least 75 percent have severe impairments, including cerebral palsy, blindness, and limited mobility. Dr. L also notes that Melanie is suffering from a serious infection, which means abortion is not a viable option. The baby will likely be born in the next 24–48 hours.

After considering this information, Melanie and her husband ask that no "extraordinary or heroic" measures be used to keep their baby alive. They specifically ask physicians to refrain from performing CPR should it be required at birth. Dr. L responds by saying that he cannot write a DNR order prior to birth, because hospital policy requires administering CPR to all infants who are born alive and weigh more than 500 grams. This policy is in place because, despite the data, prenatal diagnosis does not reliably predict outcomes for specific infants, some of whom defy the odds by surviving with little or no significant impairments. Dr. L assures the couple that, once the child is stabilized and assessed, they will have the authority to determine whether further interventions are administered. The couple reiterates their desire for a DNR order.

Less than 24 hours later, Baby S is born. Her actual birth weight is 615 grams, and she requires resuscitation. Four days after birth she suffers a brain hemorrhage, common in premature infants, which causes massive neurological damage. Baby S remains in acute care facilities for more than six months, requiring numerous additional interventions to treat emerging medical problems. When she is discharged to her parent's care, she is blind, deaf, and has significant mental and physical disabilities; it is estimated that she will not be able to walk, talk, or have meaningful interaction with those around her. She could live for many years with proper care.

Melanie and her husband sue, charging that their right to authorize treatment was usurped by the hospital, resulting in significant harm to Baby S, and significant hardship to them, not least of which will be life-long expenses for medical and personal care for their child.

Questions

1. Should parents have the right to obtain a DNR order prior to birth? If not, why? If so, subject to what restrictions?
2. Should parents have the right to obtain a DNR after birth? If not, why? If so, subject to what restrictions?
3. Should the hospital in this case be liable for damages that result from providing CPR against the parent's wishes?
4. What limits, if any, should hospitals be allowed to place on parental decision-making authority for imperiled newborns?

Resources

Annas, George. "Extremely Preterm Birth and Parental Authority to Refuse Treatment: The Case of Sidney Miller." *New England Journal of Medicine* 351, no. 20 (2004): 2118–23.

Robertson, John. "Extreme Prematurity and Parental Rights after Baby Doe." *Hastings Center Report* 34, no. 4 (2004): 32–39.

Woods, Michael. "Overriding Parental Decision to Withhold Treatment." *Virtual Mentor* 5, no. 8 (2003): 247–50. doi: 10.1001/virtualmentor.2003.5.8.hlaw1-0308.

Reference

Adapted from Woods, Michael. "Overriding Parental Decision to Withhold Treatment." *Virtual Mentor* 5, no. 8 (2003): 247–50. doi: 10.1001/virtualmentor.2003.5.8.hlaw1-0308.

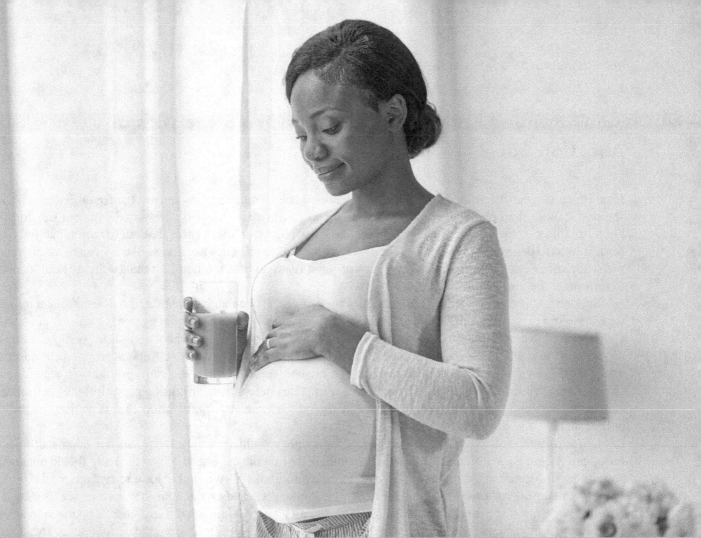

CHAPTER 3

Reproductive Ethics

3.1 Obtaining Abortion Medication in a State with an Abortion Ban

Keywords: abortion, cost of care, telemedicine

Josie B is a 19-year-old student at a large state school. Josie attended a party during the first week of class and she drank more than planned. She wakes up the next day in a strange bed with a male student she does not know, unable to remember how she got there. She is distraught, as she is careful about her sexual activity, and finds it hard to believe she would consent to sex with a person she does not know. She is even more distraught when she misses her next period, as she is clearly not ready to be a mother. She makes the difficult decision to terminate the pregnancy.

Securing abortion services is not easy, as Josie lives in a state that has instituted a near-total ban on abortion, allowing exceptions only when a woman's life is in danger or when pregnancy poses a risk of "substantial and irreversible impairment of major bodily function." The nearest legal abortion clinic is more than 400 miles away, and she lacks the means to travel, so she decides to pursue a self-managed, medical abortion, using the FDA-approved drugs mifepristone and misoprostol. Although the state prohibits in-state doctors from writing prescriptions for these drugs and out-of-state doctors from providing prescriptions via telehealth and mail services, Josie discovers a European reproductive health organization that is willing to provide online support and dispense the medication by mail.

Unfortunately, Josie's decision is complicated when her roommate, Sandy, overhears her Zoom call with the European doctor. Sandy thinks it is wrong to terminate the pregnancy, asserting that the baby should not have to pay for her drinking too much and being careless. She also thinks it's wrong for Josie to circumvent the pro-life law by "smuggling in" drugs from another country. Worse yet, Sandy points out that Josie might be subject to criminal penalties if she is caught after terminating her pregnancy. Although the law specifies punishments only for abortion providers, not for women who receive abortions, some politicians and local prosecutors are suggesting that women who induce their own abortions are essentially abortion providers. They believe prosecuting women who obtain medications via mail will send a message that their state is serious about its abortion ban.

Josie is scared by the prospect of punishment, and she is also worried about whether she could find a doctor to help in the unlikely event that she experiences complications. But she decides to proceed with her plan to terminate.

Questions

1. Do you agree with Sandy's claim that it is wrong for Josie to terminate her pregnancy in this case? If not, why? If yes, do you think Sandy should report Josie to try to prevent the abortion?

2. Do you think states should place any limits access to abortion? If not, why? If so, what kind of limits do you think should be enacted and how should they be enforced?

3. Some states allow lawsuits or criminal action against persons who "aid and abet" in abortions, including physicians, drivers, and even women who go out of state for abortion services. Do you think these penalties are justified in states with abortion bans?

4. Roe v. Wade asserted that, prior to fetal viability, access to abortion is protected by the constitutional right to privacy. Do you agree with that claim?

Resources

Belluck, Pam. "Abortion Pills Take the Spotlight as States Impose Abortion Bans." *The New York Times*, June 26, 2022.

Paul II, Pope John. "The Unspeakable Crime of Abortion." In *Evangelium Vitae,* March 25, 1995. Sections 58–62. https://www.vatican.va/content/john-paul-ii/en/encyclicals/documents/hf_jp-ii_enc_25031995_evangelium-vitae.html

Thomson, Judith Jarvis. "A Defense of Abortion." *Philosophy and Public Affairs* 1, no. 1 (1971): 47–66.

3.2 Access to Treatment for an Early Term Miscarriage

Keywords: abortion, maternal health

Dr. L works as an OB-GYN in a rural area of the southern United States, at a practice that provides mostly prenatal and maternity care. The recent Supreme Court ruling on Dobbs v. Jackson Women's Health Organization has put into effect a "trigger law" in her state, which bans abortions except when a woman's life is in danger and makes it a felony to provide women with drugs that could cause an abortion.

Dr. L sees a patient, Martha G, a few days after the trigger law takes effect. Martha is in the office for her first-trimester ultrasound. Martha and her husband Tim have been trying to get pregnant for a little over a year, and Dr. L has come to know Martha fairly well. She's almost eight weeks along with her first pregnancy and she and Tim are excited to be parents. They have already started setting up a nursery, and Tim's mother is even planning a baby shower. As Dr. L performs the ultrasound, however, she hears no heartbeat and recognizes the signs of fetal demise. She breaks the news to Tim and Martha, who are distraught. Both want to know what happened, and Dr. L has few helpful answers. She explains early pregnancy loss happens in about 10 percent of known pregnancies, and that in about a half of those cases, the fetus fails to develop properly. She assures Tim and Martha that they did not do anything wrong.

When the couple asks what to do next, Dr. L explains that there are three options. The first option is to induce miscarriage by using a combination of two drugs, mifepristone and misoprostol, which have been approved by the FDA for early pregnancy termination. The second option is to empty the contents of Martha's uterus through a surgical procedure known as dilation and curettage. The third option is to wait for a spontaneous miscarriage, which can take several weeks, and which does not occur in as many as 20 percent of cases. After some brief discussion, Martha chooses the first option, since it will allow her to plan and experience the miscarriage in the privacy of her own home and get it over with as soon as possible. It is also less invasive and much less expensive than the surgical procedure which, though very safe, has a small chance of complications, such as infection and uterine scarring.

Dr. L knows that many providers have stopped prescribing mifepristone and misoprostol after the trigger law went into effect, in order to avoid any perception that they are facilitating illegal abortions. But she writes the prescription anyway, assuming that no reasonable interpretation of the law would equate facilitating the miscarriage of a dead fetus with abortion. Martha goes straight to the pharmacy, eager to begin the process. Unfortunately, the pharmacist informs her that he cannot fill the prescription, as they no longer carry "abortion drugs." Martha soon discovers that the only other nearby pharmacy has also discontinued carrying the medications. The nearest pharmacy that carries the drugs is 100 miles away. When Martha arrives at the pharmacy with her prescription the next day, she is told that they require a confirmation from her doctor that the fetus no longer has a heartbeat, and they will need to use this documentation to get approval from the corporate office before they can dispense, a process that will take at least another day. Though sympathetic to Martha's plight, the pharmacist explains that they need to be careful not to "aid and abet" in an unlawful abortion.

Martha returns home and experiences vaginal bleeding later that night. She views this as the start of a spontaneous miscarriage, eliminating the need for another trip to retrieve the medications. But the process is not easy. After seven days of heavy bleeding, she develops a fever, and her husband takes her to the hospital, where she undergoes surgery to clear the remaining contents of her uterus, but only after the attending physicians run tests to confirm that her fetus is in fact dead.

Questions

1. Defenders of laws prohibiting abortion argue that these laws do not prohibit induced miscarriage when the fetus is dead, and that restricting access to care for miscarriage results from pharmacies and doctors who are overcautious at the expense of their patients. In contrast, many providers argue that the laws themselves are creating barriers to effective care. What is your assessment of this debate?

2. In the wake of laws banning abortion, many women who suffer miscarriages have reported difficulty accessing medications and surgical procedures that are associated with abortion. What steps might be taken to address this problem?

Resources

Belluck, Pam. "They Had Miscarriages, and New Abortion Laws Obstructed Treatment." *The New York Times*, July 17, 2022.

Harris, Lisa H. "Navigating Loss of Abortion Services — A Large Academic Medical Center Prepares for the Overturn of *Roe v. Wade*." *New England Journal of Medicine* 386, no. 22 (2022): 2061–64. https://doi.org/10.1056/NEJMp2206246.

Ollove, Michael. "Critics Fear Abortion Bans Could Jeopardize Health of Pregnant Women." *Stateline*, An Initiative of the PEW Charitable Trusts. June 22, 2022. https://pew.org/39I7iGB.

3.3 Abortion to Protect a Woman's Health: How Sick is "Sick Enough"?

Keywords: abortion, cost of care, maternal health

Alice B is 23 years old and is about 14 weeks into her second pregnancy. Her first pregnancy ended in a miscarriage at 10 weeks, leaving her and her husband Clyde deeply disappointed. The couple very much want to be parents, and they were relieved when their ultrasound at 10 weeks showed no fetal abnormalities.

Unfortunately, Alice experiences a significant vaginal discharge of fluids, and she is seeing her OB-GYN, Dr. P, for an assessment. Dr. P determines that Alice has lost amniotic fluid due to a premature rupture in her membranes, and the prognosis is grim. When a woman's "water breaks" this early, the fetus has little chance of making it to age of viability (about 24 weeks), and even less chance of being born without significant abnormalities. In most cases, women experience a spontaneous miscarriage within two weeks, though the process sometimes takes longer, and the longer it takes the greater the chance of complications.

Alice and Clyde ask whether it is possible to terminate the pregnancy to avoid the possibility of complications. Dr. P responds that this is no longer possible in their state, which has recently adopted an abortion ban. The new law only allows abortions in cases where the woman's life is at stake, or in which she faces "substantial and irreversible impairment of major bodily function." He explains that they can only perform an abortion when the fetus no longer has a heartbeat, or if Alice becomes gravely ill as a result of the pregnancy. If they want an abortion now, they will have to travel to another state. If they decide to pursue this option, he says, they should do so as soon as possible to avoid the risk of miscarriage in transit. Dr. P says he cannot make a referral to an out-of-state provider, because it might be construed as violation of the law, so they will need to do their own research if they decide to go this route.

Alice and Clyde decide that travelling for an abortion is too costly and risky, and they decide to return home to await signs of miscarriage. Within a week, Alice begins experiencing vaginal bleeding accompanied by pain and a mild fever. She returns to Dr. P, who examines her and performs an ultrasound, which determines that the fetus still has a heartbeat. He prescribes antibiotics and tells Alice to call him immediately if her condition worsens. Clyde is clearly irritated by this plan of care, asking "How sick does my wife have to get before you will perform an abortion?" Dr. P says that this is not an easy question to answer. The infection, though serious, does not yet pose a threat to Alice's life or long-term health, which means he would likely be violating the law if he performed an abortion now. Though he does not say it, Dr. P is also worried about a reporting mechanism in the new law, which provides up to $20,000 to persons who report a person who "aids and abets" in an abortion. He knows there are several staff persons in the office who are vocally "pro-life," including a nurse who recently told him about a case in which a woman whose membranes ruptured at 13 weeks went on bed rest and delivered a "miracle baby" at 26 weeks.

Ten days later, Alice returns to the office after continued bleeding and a temperature over 100 degrees. Dr. P decides to perform an abortion, based on concerns about the possibility of sepsis and damage to her uterus. He wants to safeguard his patient's health, but he worries that Alice still might not be "sick enough" under the law and he wonders what the outcome will be if he is reported by one of his staff members.

Questions

1. If you were in Dr. P's position, would you have handled this case differently? If so, how?
2. How should doctors respond when abortion laws require them to act in ways that are contrary to established standards of care and that potentially compromise their patient's health? Do doctors have an ethical duty to violate the law when it compromises the health of their patients?
3. In states that allow abortion only to protect a woman's life or health, how should the law address the question of when a woman is "sick enough" to qualify for an abortion? Does prevention of "substantial and irreversible impairment of major bodily function" provide appropriate parameters and guidance for physicians? If not, what alternative would you propose?
4. Do you think laws that reward persons for reporting illegal abortions are justified?

Resources

Arey, Whitney, Klaira Lerma, Anitra Beasley, Lorie Harper, Ghazeleh Moayedi, and Kari White. "A Preview of the Dangerous Future of Abortion Bans — Texas Senate Bill 8." *New England Journal of Medicine* 387, no. 5 (2022): 388–90. Doi: 10.1056/NEJMp2207423

Harris, Lisa H. "Navigating Loss of Abortion Services — A Large Academic Medical Center Prepares for the Overturn of *Roe v. Wade.*" *New England Journal of Medicine* 386, no. 22 (2022): 2061–64. https://doi.org/10.1056/NEJMp2206246.

Wynia, Matthew K. "Professional Civil Disobedience: Medical-Society Responsibilities after Dobbs." *New England Journal of Medicine,* NEJM.org (2022). Doi: 10.1056/NEJMp2210192

Zernike, Kate. "Medical Impact of Roe Reversal Goes Well Beyond Abortion Clinics, Doctors Say." *The New York Times*, September 10, 2022.

3.4 Abortion for an Intellectually Disabled Patient

Keywords: abortion, capacity, consent, disability, mental illness

A 17-year-old teenager, Carrie T, with previous admissions to the Crisis Unit, enters the psychiatric residential facility with symptoms of depression, suicidal ideation, and psychosis. Carrie has a history of addiction to cocaine and at times turned to prostitution to support her drug habit. During one month of individual and group treatment she is considered manipulative and frequently feigns symptoms, seeking attention. Carrie's IQ, previously tested, is 65. Although interpretation of IQ scores is controversial, scores below 70 are typically interpreted as indicating mild intellectual disability. Serving as ex-officio guardian is her grandmother, Elsa T. Tests confirm pregnancy at about three months. Carrie does not know the man responsible.

A general assessment by her physicians concludes that she is not mentally fit to be a parent. Her mental disability is compounded by her addiction and medications. Doctors consider her hazardous to the fetus. Additionally, Carrie is currently taking haloperidol to manage her mental illnesses, which has been linked with limb reduction in fetuses. Some of the staff recommend abortion. Her grandmother concurs, believing that the pregnancy is not in her granddaughter's interest and that the baby will not thrive. In addition, Elsa is not eager to take on the role of a foster mother, living sparsely herself. No other family is known.

Carrie prefers not to abort the pregnancy, but she is not adamantly opposed. She tends to agree with the doctors' advice, but is often not compliant with medical recommendations.

Questions

1. Is abortion ethically justified in this case?
2. Is Carrie's consent to an abortion sufficiently informed and voluntary? If not, what steps might be taken to address the issue?
3. Suppose Carrie was more severely disabled and lacked mental capacity to make her own medical decisions. Should an abortion be permitted based on the request and consent of her legal proxy?
4. Suppose Carrie opposed abortion. What steps, if any, should be taken to address concerns about her behaviors that are hazardous to the fetus?

Resources

Baddeley, Sarah. "Guardianship and the Abortion: A Model for Decision-Making Note." *Journal of Health & Biomedical Law* 9, no. 3 (2013): 493–520.

McCaman, Elizabeth Ann. "Limitations on Choice: Abortion for Women with Diminished Capacity." *Hastings Women's Law Journal* 24, no. 1 (2013): 155–76.

Peralta, Eyder. "Retired Massachusetts Judge Defends Forced Abortion Ruling." *NPR*, February 21, 2012, sec. America. https://www.npr.org/sections/thetwo-way/2012/02/21/147214974/retired-massachusetts-judge-defends-forced-abortion-ruling.

Reference

Adapted from Veatch, Robert M., Amy M. Haddad, and Dan English. *Case Studies in Biomedical Ethics: Decision-making, Principles, and Cases.* 2nd ed., 214. New York: Oxford University Press, 2015.

3.5 Prenatal Decisions concerning a Severely Impaired Fetus

Keywords: abortion, disability, genetic screening, impaired infants, maternal health

Trisha Y is 20 years old and six months pregnant with her first child. At her 20-week ultrasound it was discovered that her fetus had numerous problems, including heart defects and brain anomaly. Her doctor, Dr. F, ordered an amniocentesis, which uncovered trisomy 13, also known as Patau syndrome. Patau syndrome is a rare chromosomal condition in which a person has an additional copy of chromosome 13 in all or some of their body's cells. This causes severe intellectual disabilities and physical abnormalities, and many babies born with this condition have heart defects and brain and spinal cord abnormalities, among other issues. Only 5–10 percent of babies born with Patau syndrome live past their first birthday.

Dr. F informs Trisha of the diagnosis and she is distraught. He explains that there are two options available to her: They can induce labor early to terminate the pregnancy, or she can deliver the child at term and palliative care can be provided until the child passes. He also explains that because of fetal abnormalities, there is a high likelihood of fetal distress during delivery, which means that a cesarean section will be required. Though common, cesarean deliveries increase the risk of complications for women in comparison to natural birth. Dr. F suggests she go home and talk with her family about the decision. They schedule another appointment for the following week.

Trisha returns the next week with her husband, Steve. Steve explains that he and Trisha are devout Evangelical Christians and are opposed to any type of abortion. He also explains that they wish for their future child to be provided with any and all care that will help extend its life and any care that would be offered to babies born without Patau syndrome. Trisha is very quiet throughout the conversation, and merely nods her head when Dr. F asks whether she agrees with Steve's explanation about how they want to proceed.

Dr. F is unsure of how to respond. He struggles with whether it is ethical to subject Trisha to a cesarean surgery if it is unlikely the resulting baby will live longer than a few months, and he is also concerned about prolonging the child's suffering once it is born. In addition, he worries that Steve may be exerting undue influence on Trisha's decision.

Questions

1. What steps, if any, should Dr. F take to address his concerns about the welfare and consent of his patient?
2. What steps, if any, should he take to address his concerns about prolonging the suffering of a severely impaired child?
3. Do you agree with the claim that abortion would be immoral in this case?
4. Do you think abortion should be legally permitted in this kind of case?

Resources

Guinan, Patrick D. "Patau Syndrome and Perinatal Decision Making." *AMA Journal of Ethics* 7, no. 5 (2005): 336–41. https://journalofethics.ama-assn.org/article/patau-syndrome-and-perinatal-decision-making-commentary-1/2005-05

McMahan, Jeff. "Preventing the Existence of People with Disabilities." In *Quality of Life and Human Difference: Genetic Testing, Health Care, and Disability,* edited by David Wasserman, Jerome Bickenbach J, and Robert Wachbroit, 142–71. Cambridge: Cambridge University Press, 2005.

Saxton, Marsha. "Why Members of the Disability Community Oppose Prenatal Diagnosis and Selective Abortion." In *Prenatal Testing and Disability Rights,* edited by Erk Parens and Adrienne Asch, 147–64. Washington, DC: Georgetown University Press, 2000.

Vehmas, Simo. "Parental Responsibility and the Morality of Selective Abortion." *Ethical Theory and Moral Practice* 5, no. 4 (2002): 463–84. https://doi.org/10.1023/A:1021367025543.

Reference

Adapted from Guinan, Patrick D. "Patau Syndrome and Perinatal Decision Making." *AMA Journal of Ethics* 7, no. 5 (2005): 336–41. https://journalofethics.ama-assn.org/article/patau-syndrome-and-perinatal-decision-making-commentary-1/2005-05

3.6 Can Having a Child be Immoral?

Keywords: abortion, genetic testing, impaired infants, religion

Caleb and Sarah G are a newly married couple in their early twenties, who have just bought a house outside New York City. They are eager to have children and plan on having a big family. At a routine exam, Sarah tells her OB-GYN, Dr. M, that they will be starting a family soon and wonders whether she has any advice to ensure a healthy pregnancy. Apart from typical advice concerning diet and physical activity, Dr. M suggests that the couple consider getting tested to see if they are carriers for Tay–Sachs disease. Though rare, Tay–Sachs is more prominent in persons of Ashkenazi Jewish descent, a heritage shared by both Caleb and Sarah. Sarah recalls hearing something about a terrible illness that afflicted children in her family several generations back, so the couple decides to have the genetic testing. Unfortunately, the tests reveal that both Sarah and Caleb are carriers, which means that their children will have a 25 percent chance of being born with Tay–Sachs disease.

When the couple meets with Dr. M to discuss the test results, she provides them with the disturbing facts about Tay–Sachs. The symptoms, which begin three to six months after birth, include: loss of vision and hearing, seizures, spasticity, muscle wasting, and, eventually, complete paralysis. There is no cure or effective treatment for the disease, which is fatal. Children typically die by the age of four, and death is painful and protracted. Dr. M also explains that once Sarah gets pregnant, a fetal blood test can be done between the 10th and 12th week of gestation to determine whether the child will be born with Tay–Sachs. If the fetus tests positive, the couple can then decide to terminate the pregnancy and try again.

Sarah and Caleb immediately reject this last suggestion, emphasizing that they are "pro-life" and would never consider having an abortion. They tell Dr. M that they intend to "leave the matter in God's hands," praying for healthy children, while doing their best to care for any of their children who might be born with Tay–Sachs.

Dr. M is a bit taken aback by this response and struggles to remain nonjudgmental. She wants to respect the couple's reproductive freedom, but she also wants to help them avoid bringing children into the world with such a terrible disease. She points out that couples who are carriers and oppose abortion have a number of options at their disposal to avoid the risk of passing on the disease to their children. These include: adoption, use of eggs or sperm from a donor, and using IVF to create and test their own embryos prior to implantation.

Sensing disapproval, Sarah quickly rejects these suggestions as well and declares: "My ancestors have known about this disease for generations, and that didn't keep them from having kids. If I knew I was going to be judged for my pro-life stance I would have skipped the carrier testing." She also points out that many states are now prohibiting abortions after 10 weeks, which means that fetal testing would be irrelevant if she happened to live there. "Why should I feel pressured into having an abortion just because I happen to live in New York?"

Questions

1. Given their family history, do Sarah and Caleb have an obligation to test to see if they are carriers?
2. Since Sarah is unwilling to terminate a pregnancy following a positive test for Tay–Sachs, would it be immoral for her to get pregnant? Why or why not? Would your reasoning change if the probability of disease for the child was 10 percent rather than 25 percent? What if it was 90 percent?
3. Do Sarah and Caleb have an obligation to adopt, use a donor, or use IVF to screen for healthy embryos, rather than risk transmitting Tay–Sachs disease to their children?
4. How, if at all, do state abortion laws affect the morality of attempting to conceive in this case? If she lived in a state that prohibits abortion for fetal impairment, would that make Sarah's decision to conceive more or less justified?

Resources

Purdy, Laura M. "Genetic Diseases: Can Having Children Be Immoral?" In *Ethical Issues in Modern Medicine,* 3rd ed., edited by John Arras, and Nancy K. Rhoden, 311–17. Mountain View: Mayfield Publishing, 1989.

Steinbock, Bonnie and Ron McClamrock. "When Is Birth Unfair to the Child?" *Hastings Center Report* 24, no. 6 (1994): 15–21.

3.7 Recruiting a Commercial Surrogate

Keywords: coercion, surrogacy

Cathy M has been employed by a large commercial surrogacy agency in California for more than two decades. Prior to working in the surrogacy industry, she was a surrogate mother herself, delivering a healthy baby boy to a happy couple. She is passionate about surrogacy and the joy it can bring to couples who are having trouble conceiving children on their own, and she is proud of her work in the industry. But she has become increasingly concerned about the practices at her company, which has been recently purchased by a large national corporation. The number of commercial surrogacy companies in California has grown, in part to meet the growing demand for surrogates, and companies are now competing for a shrinking pool of surrogates. In order to meet market demand, some companies have started to loosen their selection criteria, by lowering the threshold by which potential surrogates can demonstrate "financial independence," and by approving women who are healthy but who score very low on screening questions that are used to determine "altruistic motivation." They have also started increasing "signing bonuses" that are provided to surrogates when they sign their legal agreement. Cathy is now assessing the application of Mary G, a 27-year-old woman who barely meets the company's financial independence criteria. Her husband has been employed at a local warehouse for many years, but the company has said layoffs are possible in the coming year, and Mary is concerned about his job security. Mary is healthy and she is not conflicted about giving up the child she will carry, to whom she will not be genetically related, but she is clearly pursuing surrogacy only because it provides her with the best opportunity to support her family. She is especially excited about the $4,000 signing bonus.

Cathy is conflicted about whether to approve Mary's application. In the past, she would not have approved an applicant in these circumstances, but the company is pressuring her to bring more surrogates on board. In addition, she believes rejecting the application would only cause Mary to apply at another firm that is likely to accept her.

Questions

1. Should Cathy approve Mary's surrogacy application?
2. Should altruistic motivation be a factor in selecting women for commercial surrogacy? How might this be measured?
3. Is there a point at which commercial surrogacy becomes exploitative of women who are suffering from financial hardship? If so, how would you make that determination?
4. What criteria should be used to determine whether a woman is a good candidate for surrogacy?
5. Should there be federal and/or state rules that must be met before a company can hire a woman to be a surrogate? If not, why? If so, what rules would you recommend?

Resources

Dodge, David. "Meet the Women Who Become Surrogates." *The New York Times*, Feb. 15, 2021.

Steinbock, Bonnie. "Surrogate Motherhood as Prenatal Adoption." *Law, Medicine, and Health Care* 16, no. 1–2 (1988): 44–50.

3.8 A Surrogate Violates the Terms of her Contract

Keywords: confidentiality, surrogacy

Valerie C is a 28-year-old mother of one who has agreed to act as a surrogate for a couple. Valerie and the couple have entered into a contract that offers Valerie compensation for her carrying the fetus to term and requires her to abstain from actions that might hurt the developing fetus, including the use of drugs and alcohol. Valerie is being paid $50,000 for being a surrogate, and she is receiving this money in monthly installments. All of Valerie's medical bills will be paid by the couple, but the couple have agreed to let Valerie choose her own doctors, as long as she reports on all prenatal visits and keeps the couple updated on the progress of the pregnancy. Valerie has chosen to work with Dr. K, the obstetrician who delivered her own daughter three years ago. Dr. K has only worked with two surrogates before, and in those instances, the contracting couples were always present at any appointments and established a relationship with Dr. K.

Valerie comes in to see Dr. K for her third prenatal visit, and her first prenatal visit in her second trimester. She reports no real problems with her pregnancy, and Dr. K confirms that all looks well. Before ending the visit, Dr. K asks if Valerie has any questions for her. Valerie looks abashed, but after a minute explains to Dr. K that it's been harder for her to give up marijuana use entirely than she thought it would be. She admits to using edible marijuana products "a few times a month" because she read online that occasional marijuana use during pregnancy was very low risk. She also indicates that small doses of edibles are helping with nausea she is experiencing due to pregnancy.

Dr. K tells Valerie that he recommends not using edibles, because the effects of marijuana on fetuses have not been widely studied. He also points out that she has violated the conditions of her surrogate contract, which might allow the couple to withhold further payments. He wonders whether he should note Valerie's marijuana use in the medical record, which the couple has a right to see as part of the agreement.

Questions

1. Should Dr. K note Valerie's admission of marijuana use in the medical record? Would this constitute a breach of confidentiality?

2. Would the couple be justified in withholding further monthly payments, pending a clean drug test by Valerie?

3. What kinds of stipulations should be allowed in surrogate contracts? Is there a point at which restrictions constitute an unjust violation of a surrogate's autonomy?

Resources

Horner, Claire and Paul Burcher. "A Surrogate's Secrets Are(n't) Safe with Me: Patient Confidentiality in the Care of a Gestational Surrogate." *Journal of Medical Ethics* 47, no. 4 (2021): 213–17. doi:10.1136/medethics-2017-104518.

Rafique, Saima and Alan H. DeCherney. "Physician Responsibility When a Surrogate Mother Breaks Her Contract." *AMA Journal of Ethics* 16, no. 1 (2014): 10–16. https://journalofethics.ama-assn.org/article/physician-responsibility-when-surrogate-mother-breaks-her-contract/2014-01

Reference

Adapted from Rafique, Saima and Alan H. DeCherney. "Physician Responsibility When a Surrogate Mother Breaks Her Contract." *AMA Journal of Ethics* 16, no. 1 (2014): 10–16. https://journalofethics.ama-assn.org/article/physician-responsibility-when-surrogate-mother-breaks-her-contract/2014-01

3.9 Surrogacy: A Disagreement over Selective Reduction and Parental Rights

Keywords: abortion, surrogacy

Deepti D is a 37-year-old mother of two from California who has entered into a surrogacy contract with contracting parents Natalie and Shane. Deepti is implanted with embryos created from eggs from Natalie and sperm from Shane. After the embryo implantation, it is discovered that Deepti is carrying triplets. Natalie and Shane are concerned, both about the risks that multiple pregnancies carry for fetuses, as well as about their ability to care for three newborns. They ask Deepti to abort one of the three fetuses through a process known as "selective reduction." Deepti is surprised and angered by the request and files a lawsuit seeking custody of one of the potential children. Alerted to the lawsuit, Natalie and Shane ask to claim parental rights over all three potential children. Deepti refuses to drop the lawsuit.

Questions

1. Should Deepti be given parental rights to the third potential child?
2. The case states that Natalie and Shane are the genetic parents, as well as the contracting parents. Assume that instead, Deepti's eggs and Shane's sperm were used to create the embryos. Does this impact your reasoning regarding who should be awarded custody of the third potential child?
3. If Deepti had signed a contract agreeing to abort fetuses at the request of the contracting parents before implantation of the embryos, would that impact your reasoning about this case?

Resources

Forman, Deborah L. "Abortion Clauses in Surrogacy Contracts: Insights from a Case Study Symposium on Assisted Reproductive Technology and Family Law." *Family Law Quarterly* 49, no. 1 (2015–2016): 29–54.

Lewin, Tamar. "Surrogates and Couples Face a Maze of Laws, State by State." *The New York Times,* September 17, 2014.

London, Catherine. "Advancing a Surrogate-Focused Model of Gestational Surrogacy Contracts." *Cardozo Journal of Law and Gender* 18, no. 2 (2012): 391–422.

3.10 Selling Eggs to a "Selective" Fertility Clinic

Keywords: coercion, eugenics, genetic testing

Michelle W is a third-year doctoral candidate in a philosophy program. She and some of her female colleagues have received emails from a local fertility clinic inquiring about their interest in donating gametes (eggs) for use by those with the money to purchase them. The clinic describes itself as "elite," catering to a wealthy clientele, and offering the best compensation to egg donors. Compensation for donation is $10,000, which is about half as much as Michelle's yearly graduate stipend pays. This money is significant to Michelle, as she is having trouble making ends meet while she pursues her graduate studies. Michelle researches the process of egg donation and learns it would take a little over a month. She would need to inject herself with hormones which would cause her body to release more eggs than it would during a normal menstrual cycle. She would have in-office appointments once a day for about 10 days, and her eggs would be gathered via a needle through vaginal tissue when they've been released. All medical expenses would be covered by the clinic. She learns that although the hormones she would need to take might cause mood swings, headaches, and some other minor side effects, most egg donors experience only short-term mild side effects. On balance, Michelle thinks the risks and inconveniences are outweighed by the compensation she will receive.

The only thing that gives Michelle a pause is the part of the reproductive medicine clinic's website aimed at potential recipients of eggs. The website emphasizes that potential parents can select gamete donors based on a variety of factors that Michelle finds problematic. In addition to gametes and gamete donors being screened for genetic diseases and other health issues, potential parents are also given access to a host of information about the donor: educational level attained, IQ scores if available, height, weight, ethnicity, race, hair color, eye color, and even significant athletic or artistic achievements. The clinic also allows prospective parents who use their IVF service to purchase additional screening of fertilized embryos. This screening tests for both negative traits, such as diseases, and positive traits, like height and cognitive ability. The company emphasizes that screening for positive traits is not yet reliable, but it believes parents who want to purchase this information should be able to do so. Their goal is to provide parents with any information that might help them have "the child of their dreams." Michelle worries about the possible eugenicist implications of the clinic's screening and testing services, and wonders whether she should instead work with another clinic in town that provides significantly less compensation.

Questions

1. Should the sale of human gametes be permitted?
2. Is Michelle right to be concerned about the "eugenicist implications" of the clinic's practices? What is wrong with providing parents with the option of genetic tests, so long as the clinic is truthful about the accuracy of these tests?
3. Do you think certain kinds of information about donors should not be provided to prospective parents? If so, where would you draw the line and why?
4. Do you think certain kinds of genetic testing should not be allowed? If so, where would you draw the line and why?

Resources

Daniels, Cynthia R., and Erin Heidt-Forsythe. "Gendered Eugenics and the Problematic of Free Market Reproductive Technologies: Sperm and Egg Donation in the United States." *Signs: Journal of Women in Culture and Society* 37, no. 3 (2012): 719–47. https://doi.org/10.1086/662964.

Kenney, Nancy and Michelle McGowan. "Egg Donation Compensation: Ethical and Legal Challenges." *Medicolegal and Bioethics* 14, no. 4 (2014): 124. https://doi.org/10.2147/MB.S51328.

Klitzman, Robert. "Buying and Selling Human Eggs: Infertility Providers' Ethical and Other Concerns Regarding Egg Donor Agencies." *BMC Medical Ethics* 17, no. 1 (2016): 71. https://doi.org/10.1186/s12910-016-0151-z.

3.11 Using IVF for a "Savior Sibling"

Keywords: cancer, IVF, pediatrics, prenatal screening

Mike and Laura G's three-year-old daughter Ella has been diagnosed with acute lymphocytic leukemia and needs a bone marrow transplant to survive. Although family members are the most likely persons to be matches, Mike, Laura, and other family members are tested and found not to be close enough matches for the bone marrow needed to treat Ella. Ella's doctor, Dr. J, talks with Mike and Laura about the possibility of having another child. She explains that by using In Vitro Fertilization (IVF) and Preimplantation Genetic Diagnosis (PGD) an embryo can be selected for implantation that is a genetic match to Ella. Umbilical cord blood and placenta can be harvested at the birth of this potential child for use in treating Ella. Mike and Laura wanted to have another child and consider whether they should use these technologies to create a "savior sibling" for Ella.

Questions

1. Would creating a savior sibling in this case compromise the welfare or dignity of the child?
2. If you object to the creation of savior siblings under any circumstance, what is the basis for your objection?
3. If you are sympathetic to the creation of a savior sibling in this case, do you think there are circumstances in which it would be wrong to create a savior sibling? If so, where would you draw those lines?

Resources

Dickens, B.M. "Preimplantation Genetic Diagnosis and 'Savior Siblings.'" *International Journal of Gynecology and Obstetrics* 88, no. 1 (2005): 91–96. https://doi.org/10.1016/j.ijgo.2004.10.002.

Rubeis, Giovanni and Florian Steger. "Saving Whom? The Ethical Challenges of Harvesting Tissue from Savior Siblings." *European Journal of Haematology* 103, no. 5 (2019): 478–82. https://doi.org/10.1111/ejh.13313.

Strong, Kimberly, Ian Kerridge, and Miles Little. "Savior Siblings, Parenting and the Moral Valorization of Children: Savior Siblings, Parenting and the Moral Valorization of Children." *Bioethics* 28, no. 4 (2014): 187–93. https://doi.org/10.1111/j.1467-8519.2012.02001.x.

3.12 Sex Selection for Family Balancing

Keywords: genetic testing, IVF, prenatal screening

Dr. S is the medical director of a busy fertility practice. She is meeting with Mary and Bill W for an IVF consultation. Mary and Bill have already had three boys via IVF, since they had trouble conceiving naturally due to Mary's blocked fallopian tubes. Dr. S is surprised to see them again because, at the time of the last pregnancy, they mentioned that finances would preclude them from having a fourth child. Now they tell her that they have reconsidered because they would like to have a daughter. If they can select only female embryos for transfer, they tell her, they would like to try again.

Dr. S is unsure how to respond to this request. She cautions them that there is extra cost and risk associated with the embryo manipulation required to determine sex. Additionally, there is always the possibility that all the embryos in the cycle will be male. The couple states that, in that case, they would not have any of the male embryos transferred, since they do not want another son. They say that they are willing to undertake the cost and invasive procedures even with the knowledge that they might not get any healthy female embryos. Dr. S tells them that she will have to discuss this request with the rest of the practice, including the embryologists, to see if all parties involved are comfortable with proceeding.

Questions

1. What are the most significant ethical concerns about using IVF for purposes of sex selection?
2. Do you think Dr. S should help this couple try to have a daughter?
3. Suppose the couple was childless and only intended to have one child, for which they want to select the sex. Would this alter your ethical assessment?
4. Is selection of specific embryos for "family balancing" ethically different from other forms of nonmedical selectivity, such as selection for physical or cognitive traits that are deemed desirable?
5. Should there be regulations restricting the use of prenatal genetic testing and selectivity? If so, what regulations do you think should be enacted?

Resources

Ethics Committee of the American Society for Reproductive Medicine. "Use of Reproductive Technology for Sex Selection for Nonmedical Reasons." *Fertility and Sterility* 117, no. 4 (2022): 720–26.

King, Louise P. "Sex Selection for Non-Medical Reasons." *AMA Journal of Ethics* 9, no. 6 (2007): 418–22. https://journalofethics.ama-assn.org/article/sex-selection-nonmedical-reasons/2007-06.

Lieman, Harry J. and Andrzej K. Breborowicz. "Sex Selection for Family Balancing." *AMA Journal of Ethics* 16, no. 10 (2014): 797–802. https://journalofethics.ama-assn.org/sites/journalofethics.ama-assn.org/files/2018-05/ecas3-1410.pdf

Reference

From Lieman, Harry J. and Andrzej K. Breborowicz. "Sex Selection for Family Balancing." *AMA Journal of Ethics* 16, no. 10 (2014): 797–802. https://journalofethics.ama-assn.org/sites/journalofethics.ama-assn.org/files/2018-05/ecas3-1410.pdf

3.13 Selecting Embryos for Deafness

Keywords: disability, eugenics, genetic testing, IVF, prenatal screening

Maddie and Ryan K are in their late twenties, and both have been deaf since their births. They come from families who adapted well to their genetic deafness, and they have lived full lives, including graduating from college and holding jobs they enjoy. Both have been actively involved in Deaf communities since they were young, and hope to have a child who can participate in and appreciate Deaf culture. They have now been married for three years, and they are ready to have a child.

Maddie and Ryan come to Dr. S's fertility clinic and explain that they want to use In Vitro Fertilization (IVF) and Preimplantation Genetic Diagnosis (PGD) in order to select an embryo that possesses congenital markers for deafness for implantation. Both Maddie and Ryan are healthy and could likely conceive without medical intervention. Dr. S has assisted many couples who use PGD to avoid having children with impairments, but he has never had clients who want to use PGD to have children with a recognized disability. He wonders what to do.

Questions

1. Should Dr. S assist this couple in their desire to have a deaf child? What factors should he consider in making this decision?

2. If you believe selectivity for deafness is permissible, would you also support selectivity for other forms of disability, such as blindness or paralysis? Why or why not?

3. Suppose the couple in this case suffered from achondroplastic dwarfism and wanted to use IVF to select a child with the same condition. Would that choice be ethically defensible?

4. How does our understanding of "disability" affect the assessment of selective reproduction in this case?

Resources

Kolthoff, Marta. "Assisted Reproduction and *Primum Non Nocere.*" *AMA Journal of Ethics* 9, no. 9 (2007): 605–10 https://journalofethics.ama-assn.org/article/assisted-reproduction-and-primum-non-nocere/2007-09

Wallis, Jacqueline Mae. "Is It Ever Morally Permissible to Select for Deafness in One's Child*?" Medicine, Health Care and Philosophy* 23 (2020): 3–15. https://doi.org/10.1007/s11019-019-09922-6

3.14 Advising a Patient about Direct-to-Consumer Prenatal Test Results

Keywords: eugenics, genetic testing, prenatal screening, veracity

Mandy R is 35 years old, and she is about 12 weeks pregnant with her first child. She and her husband are excited, as they have been trying to conceive unsuccessfully for several years. But Mandy's excitement is tempered by the knowledge that, due to her age, she has a higher risk of having a child with a genetic disorder. In fact, her cousin recently had a child with Down Syndrome at age 36. She is not sure she would continue a pregnancy if she discovered her fetus had a serious disorder, so she searches online for information about genetic testing. She quickly discovers several Direct-to-Consumer (DTC) companies that offer noninvasive tests, which only require her to submit a blood sample at a local lab. A representative for one of these companies informs her that her insurance will pay not only for Down Syndrome screening, but for a number of less common but very serious diseases that result from chromosomal abnormalities. Mandy is delighted to hear this. She consents to all the tests and submits her blood sample.

Ten days later, Mandy receives troubling news. Although the test for Down Syndrome was negative, her test was positive for Prader–Willi syndrome, a rare disorder that causes serious physical, mental, and behavioral disorders throughout life. Mandy is devastated by this news. After several tearful days and restless nights, she is finally able to get in to see her gynecologist, Dr. H, to discuss how to proceed.

Dr. H barely glances at the test results before setting them aside and telling Mandy that he wishes she had consulted him before ordering the tests, because he could have spared her a lot of heartache. He says DTC noninvasive tests are very accurate for Down Syndrome, but notoriously unreliable for rare conditions such as Prader–Willi. For these conditions, positive tests can be wrong about 90 percent of the time. Mandy is surprised by this news, noting that the company website featured claims about reliable and accurate results, with no mention of false positives. "That's all marketing," says Dr. H, "they do it because the law allows it, and they know people fall for that stuff." The good news, he says, is that her baby probably doesn't have either Down Syndrome or Prader–Willi. But to confirm the absence of Prader–Willi, Mandy would need to undergo amniocentesis, a more invasive test that involves a very small risk of miscarriage. Dr. H also mentions that this additional test is more costly than the noninvasive blood screening and it may not be covered by her insurance. He says the decision to have the additional testing is entirely up to her. If she had come to him ahead of time, he may have recommended amnio for Down Syndrome later in pregnancy, but not for Prader–Willi or other rare conditions. And he would have definitely advised against buying tests for rare conditions from DTC companies that are "only in it to make a buck." He tells Mandy she could just ignore the positive test result, knowing it is almost always incorrect, or she could undergo the additional testing to put her mind at ease. He asks her what she wants to do.

Mandy is unsure how to proceed and says she will have to think about it. She was hoping for more definitive advice from Dr. H, who she feels has been a bit judgmental and not very supportive.

Questions

1. Do you think Mandy should undergo the additional testing? What factors should she consider in making this decision?
2. Do you think Dr. H provided Mandy with sufficient guidance and support? If not, what do you think he should have done differently?
3. Do you think companies that sell DTC prenatal testing should be subject to government regulation? If so, what rules and requirements do you think should be placed on such companies?
4. Some countries prohibit any kind of DTC genetic testing, including ancestry tests, and only allow doctors to order genetic testing for their patients. Would you support such a ban? Why or why not?

Resources

American College of Obstetricians and Gynecologists. "Committee Opinion No. 816: Consumer Testing for Disease Risk." *Obstetrics and Gynecology* 137, no. 1 (2021): E1–6. https://www.acog.org/clinical/clinical-guidance/committee-opinion/articles/2021/01/consumer-testing-for-disease-risk

Brothers, Kyle B. and Esther E. Knapp. "How Should Primary Care Physicians Respond to Direct-to-Consumer Genetic Test Results?" *AMA Journal of Ethics* 20, no. 9 (2018): E812–18. https://journalofethics.ama-assn.org/article/how-should-primary-care-physicians-respond-direct-consumer-genetic-test-results/2018-09

Kliff, Sarah and Aatish Bhatia, "When They Warn of Rare Disorders, These Prenatal Tests Are Usually Wrong." *The New York Times,* January 1, 2022. https://www.nytimes.com/2022/01/01/upshot/pregnancy-birth-genetic-testing.html

Schaper, Manuel and Silkie Shicktanz. "Medicine, Market, and Communication: Ethical Considerations in regard to Persuasive Communication in Direct-to-Consumer Genetic Testing Services." *BMC Medical Ethics* 19 (2018): 56. https://doi.org/10.1186/s12910-018-0292-3

3.15 Fringe Benefits for Family Planning

Keywords: veracity

Megan H is a 32-year-old woman who recently got her dream job at Techtropolis, one of the biggest information technology companies in the country. When she is at orientation, a representative from human resources offers a presentation on the company's health care benefits. Megan is surprised to learn that Techtropolis offers generous family planning benefits, including up to $20,000 for Oocyte Cryopreservation (OCP), commonly known as "egg freezing." The HR rep tells Megan that this benefit is intended to promote reproductive choice, by allowing women to work longer before having kids, if they decide that is best for them. In addition, Techtropolis offers 18 weeks of paid maternity leave, with an option for 6 additional weeks without pay. The HR rep notes that this goes well beyond federal law, which only requires companies to offer 12 weeks of unpaid maternity leave. These benefits are attractive to Megan, since she and her husband Mario want to have kids. The egg freezing benefit is especially intriguing, since she would like to get a few years under her belt at Techtropolis before having a child, and she is worried that her "biological clock" is ticking.

When Megan discusses these family planning benefits with Mario, he too is pleasantly surprised. But he is a little skeptical about egg freezing, which he says, "sounds too good to be true." He also wonders whether Techtropolis is more concerned about keeping female employees on the job than promoting reproductive choice. After Mario expresses these concerns, Megan goes online to gather more information on OCP, and she is amazed at the number of websites for fertility clinics offering OCP. A typical website asserts that thousands of women are using OCP "to extend their child-bearing window" and "increase career choices," and provides testimonials from women who felt "empowered, relieved, and in charge of their future" after undergoing OCP. It also has links to "success stories" of women who have had children via OCP. While she appreciates Mario's skepticism, she is starting to think that OCP might be a good option for her.

Questions

1. What factors should Megan consider in determining whether OCP is the right choice for her?
2. Do you agree with the claim that companies promote reproductive freedom for female employees by paying for OCP?
3. Many large corporations are starting to cover OCP in their benefits, and clinics offering OCP services are increasing. What are the most significant ethical concerns associated with the growing use of OCP? Do you think these concerns justify restricting the use of OCP? If so, how?
4. Federally mandated family leave is far less in the United States in comparison to other countries. Should federally mandated family leave in the United States be increased? What are the advantages and disadvantages of family leave policies in other countries in comparison to the United States?

Resources

American Society for Reproductive Medicine. "Planned Oocyte Cryopreservation for Women Seeking to Preserve Future Reproductive Potential: An Ethics Committee Opinion." *Fertility and* Sterility 110, no. 6 (2018): 1022–28. https://doi.org/10.1016/j.fertnstert.2018.08.027

La Ferla, Ruth. "These Companies Really, Really, Really Want to Freeze Your Eggs." *The New York Times,* August 29, 2018. https://www.nytimes.com/2018/08/29/style/egg-freezing-fertility-millennials.html

Pacia, Danielle and Jacob Howard. "Surprising Surge of Egg Freezing during the Pandemic Raises Ethical Questions." *Hastings Center Bioethics Forum.* January 21, 2021. https://www.thehastingscenter.org/surprising-surge-of-egg-freezing-during-the-pandemic-raises-ethical-questions/

Pflum, Mary. "Egg Freezing 'Startups' Have Wall Street Talking—and Traditional Fertility Doctors Worried." *NBC News,* March 4, 2019. https://www.nbcnews.com/health/features/egg-freezing-start-ups-have-wall-street-talking-traditional-fertility-doctors-n978526

3.16　Assisted Reproduction for an Older Couple

Keywords: IVF, paternalism

Carly L is a 53-year-old corporate executive who has been happily married to Dan for almost 30 years. Dan is 62 years old, but their age gap has never been an issue and they are both in good health. Dan is the head of a successful engineering firm, which he has worked hard to build over the time of their marriage. Carly and Dan have always wanted kids, but they decided to postpone parenthood because of the demands of their careers. When Carly was 26 and Dan was 34, they decided to freeze their gametes for future use, so they could become parents of their own biological child "when the time was right." That time is now, since Dan is nearing retirement and Carly is at a stage of her career where she can delegate duties, which means they will both have plenty of time to enjoy raising a child.

Carly and Dan visit Dr. P, a well-known fertility specialist, to inquire about starting the process of assisted reproduction. This will involve using IVF to fertilize Carly's eggs with Dan's sperm, and then implanting up to two embryos in her uterus. The hope is at least one egg will take, allowing Carly to carry a child to term. Dr. P is meeting the couple for the first time, and he is impressed by their careful family planning and their overall good health. But Carly and Dan are much older than most persons who seek help at his clinic, and he has some concerns about their age. At 53, Carly will face slightly higher risks of complications during pregnancy, but these are not significant enough to cause Dr. P concern, as long as Carly understands these risks. His main concerns are social. By the time their child starts high school, Carly will be nearly 70 and Dan will be approaching 80. This age gap might present numerous parenting challenges. More obviously, their child will have an increased chance of losing one or even both parents before the age of 18 or could have to provide care for aged and ill parents early in life. Though there are no federal and few state laws that set age limits for assisted reproduction, many fertility clinics will not implant eggs in women over 50, and some surrogate agencies impose a combined age limit of 108 on intended parents. Similarly, adoption agencies often refuse adoptions for couples in their 50s, preferring to place children with younger couples, or impose a "40-year rule," which limits the age gap between adopted children and their parents. These age limits are all in place to protect the welfare of children.

Dr. P explains that this is his first time working with a couple over 50 and, noting the age limits imposed by some adoption and fertility agencies, says he would like to consult with his colleagues before deciding how to proceed with their case.

Carly and Dan are surprised and somewhat irate when Dr. P expresses these concerns. Carly declares that she is better prepared to be a mom now than she was in her 30s, and she suggests that the policies described by Dr. P are "blatantly ageist." She declares: "If I withheld benefits from employees based on their age, I'd probably find myself in court!"

Questions

1. Should Dr. P help Carly get pregnant?
2. Suppose Carly's husband was 32 rather than 62, or suppose Carly was single. Would those variations affect your reasoning about the morality of reproduction in this case?
3. Is it "ageist" for fertility clinics, surrogate agencies, and adoption agencies to privilege younger persons by placing limits on the age of prospective parents?
4. Is age relevant to morally responsible procreation? Is there an age at which it would be immoral to have children?
5. In what ways might the welfare of children be compromised by having older parents? In what ways might children benefit from having older parents?

Resources

Ethics Committee of the American Society for Reproductive Medicine. "Oocyte or Embryo Donation to Women of Advanced Reproductive Age: An Ethics Committee Opinion." *Fertility and Sterility* 106, no. 5 (2016): e3–7. http://dx.doi.org/10.1016/j.fertnstert.2016.07.002

Fisseha, Senait and Natalie A. Clark. "Assisted Reproduction for Postmenopausal Women." *AMA Journal of Ethics* 16, no. 1 (2014): 5–9. https://journalofethics.ama-assn.org/article/assisted-reproduction-post-menopausal-women/2014-01

3.17 A Woman's Request for Tubal Ligation is Denied

Keywords: autonomy, paternalism, sterilization

Kim B is a 23-year-old woman who has recently graduated college and started her first job at a law firm. Kim had a difficult childhood, as she and her two siblings were abused and neglected by their parents. Kim worked hard in school to achieve independence, and she long ago decided that she did not want to have children. She is haunted by the specter of her abusive childhood and worries that she might not be a good parent. She is also worried about the history of alcoholism in her family. Both her parents were active alcoholics, and she is five years sober after struggling with binge drinking in her teens. Family issues aside, Kim believes having children would interfere with her desire to advance in her law career. She is also tired of using birth control, and dreads the possibility of an accidental pregnancy, since access to abortion is extremely limited in her state. Considering all these factors, Kim decides to see her doctor to request a tubal ligation, which will prevent her from having kids.

Kim visits Dr. T, her gynecologist, and explains the various reasons for her request for a tubal ligation. Dr. T listens patiently, before stating that he does not perform tubal ligations on women who are under 30, unmarried, or have never had children. He explains that tubal ligation is an irreversible procedure, and in his experience women's views on having kids sometimes change. In fact, he says a recent study shows that 20 percent of women under 30 who have the procedure regret doing so. On a more personal level, Dr. T points out that coming from an abusive family does not mean Kim would be a bad mother, and he believes her concerns about alcoholism in the family are unwarranted. Alcoholism, he says, is not primarily about genetics but family environment, and the important thing is that she no longer drinks. Instead of tubal ligation, he recommends continued contraception, which will allow Kim preserve the possibility of having children if her circumstances should change. "Suppose you fall in love with someone who wants to have children," he says, "sterilization could be a sticking point in an otherwise wonderful relationship."

Kim is a little taken aback by Dr. T's comments, and she is especially irritated by his last remark. She knows the doctor has a duty to be sure she understands the implications of the procedure, but she thinks he's getting a little too personal and paternalistic. Why can't he just respect her decision?

Kim resolves to visit another gynecologist, but she worries that the path to tubal ligation might be more difficult than she envisioned.

Questions

1. Is Dr. T's refusal to provide tubal ligation surgery for Kim paternalistic? Do you think this refusal is justified?
2. Do you think Dr. T does a good job explaining the implications of tubal ligation to Kim? If not, what do you think he should have done differently?
3. Do physicians who perform tubal ligations have an ethical obligation to provide them to all women who offer voluntary and informed consent?
4. Do you think doctors who refuse requests for tubal ligation from women who are under 30, unmarried, and without children should also refuse requests from similarly situated men who want vasectomies?

Resources

American College of Obstetricians and Gynecologists. "Committee Opinion No. 695: Sterilization of Women: Ethical Issues and Considerations." *Obstetrics and Gynecology* 129, no. 4 (2017): E109–16. https://www.acog.org/clinical/clinical-guidance/committee-opinion/articles/2017/04/sterilization-of-women-ethical-issues-and-considerations

Cunha, Darlena. "The Outrageous Reasons These Women Couldn't Get Their Tubes Tied." *Vice,* May 7, 2019. https://www.vice.com/en/article/9kxam7/tubal-ligation-requirements-doctor-denials

McGowan, Emma. "Can Doctors Refuse Tubal Ligation? Here's Why It's Hard to Get One." *Bustle,* October 21, 2019. https://www.bustle.com/life/can-i-get-my-tubes-tied-process-for-tubal-ligation

Tazkargy, Ariel S. "From Coercion to Coercion: Voluntary Sterilization Policies in the United States." *Minnesota Journal of Law and Inequality* 32, no. 1 (2014): 135–68. https://scholarship.law.umn.edu/lawineq/vol32/iss1/5

3.18 Request to Sterilize an Intellectually Disabled Girl

Keywords: consent, disability, paternalism, sterilization, surrogate decision-making

Myra D is 16 years old, and she is intellectually disabled. Her disability is classified as moderate to severe, based on an assessed IQ of 40. Myra lives with her parents, Adam and Beverly, who work hard to provide everything she needs, which is no small task. Myra has had a combination of home schooling and special education. Her ability to communicate with and understand others is very limited, and she has learned to do some but not all of her daily self-care tasks. In addition to school, she has been able to engage in limited activities outside the home. These include walking to the store two blocks from her house to buy candy and participating in activities at a community center that sponsors events for disabled citizens. These outside activities are beneficial for Myra and also give her parents much needed breaks from their care-giving duties.

As Myra has grown, her sexual development has created challenges. She has difficulty managing menstrual periods, which is a source of significant stress for both her and her parents. She has also become sexually interested, as indicated by her attempt touch a boy's genitals during an event at the community center. Myra's parents are now wary of letting her go to the store by herself, as they have read that children with intellectual disabilities are up to five times more likely to be sexually abused. They are also concerned about the possibility of pregnancy which, though remote, would have devastating consequences for their family. Myra is obviously unfit to be a parent, and her parents lack the financial, emotional, and physical means to care for another child. An abortion would be difficult if not impossible to acquire in their state.

Adam and Beverly bring Myra to a local clinic to solicit advice about how to handle this challenge. They are assigned to Dr. G, a new physician who is handling gynecology cases at the clinic. Dr. G tells them that the simplest solution is to put Myra on oral contraceptives. Continuous contraceptives would suppress menstruation and would also prevent pregnancy. Dr. G says the pills are generally considered safe, but some studies have linked long-term use to a small increase in the risk of breast cancer, blood clots, and stroke. Adam and Beverly express concern over this last point. Nondisabled women might assume these risks because they want to preserve fertility while being sexually active, but neither of these applies to Myra. They also wonder whether it will be feasible to have her swallow pills every day until menopause, as she is not always cooperative about taking medications. Beverly asks, "Wouldn't my daughter's interests be best served by performing a hysterectomy? Can you help us get the process started for that?"

Dr. G is unsure how to respond to this request. She knows sterilization is sometimes performed on disabled persons, but she also knows it is highly controversial. She tells Adam and Beverly she will need to discuss their request with colleagues and asks them to schedule a return visit for the following week.

Questions

1. What factors should Dr. G consider in determining whether to support the request to perform a hysterectomy on Myra? Do you think she should support this request? If not, what alternative should she recommend?

2. What are the most significant ethical concerns associated with sterilization of persons with intellectual disabilities? Under what circumstances, if any, do you believe sterilization of intellectually disabled persons should be permitted?

3. State laws vary with respect to sterilization of persons with intellectual disabilities. They range from prohibiting sterilization without informed consent, to allowing it without patient consent at the request of a parent or medical professional. Among those that allow sterilization, some require court approval, but others do not. What legal requirements do you think should govern sterilization of persons with intellectual disabilities?

Resources

American College of Obstetricians and Gynecologists. "Committee Opinion No. 695: Sterilization of Women: Ethical Issues and Considerations." *Obstetrics and Gynecology* 129, no. 4 (2017): E109–16. https://www.acog.org/clinical/clinical-guidance/committee-opinion/articles/2017/04/sterilization-of-women-ethical-issues-and-considerations

Denekins, Joke, Herman Nys, and Hugo Stuer. "Sterilization of incompetent Mentally Handicapped Persons: A Model for Decision-making." *Journal of Medical Ethics* 25, no. 3 (1999): 237–41. http://dx.doi.org/10.1136/jme.25.3.237

Kamenev, Marina. "Sterilizing a Child, for a Better Life." *The Atlantic*, September 19, 2013. https://www.theatlantic.com/health/archive/2013/09/sterilizing-a-child-for-a-better-life/279765/

Reiter, Jesse. "Involuntary Sterilization of Disabled Americans: An Historical Overview." *ABC Law Centers*, November 6, 2018. https://www.abclawcenters.com/blog/2018/11/06/involuntary-sterilization-of-disabled-americans-an-historical-overview/

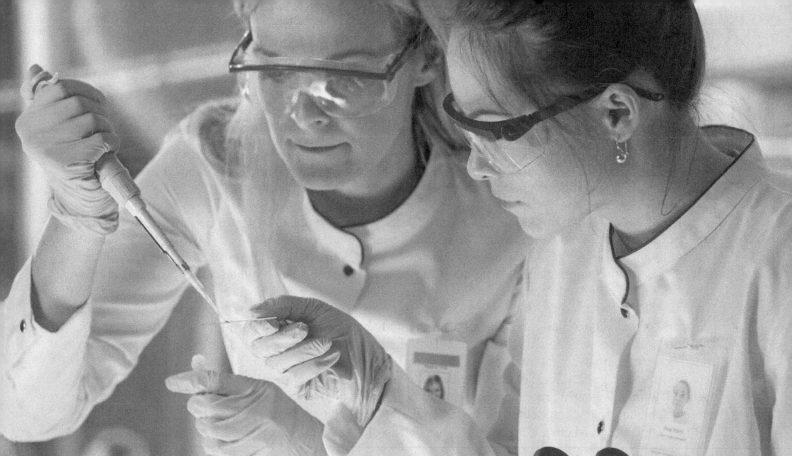

CHAPTER **4**

Research and Technologies

4.1 Using Nazi Data

Keywords: consent, human subject research, prisoners

Andrew H is a professor of philosophy at a research university who specializes in biomedical ethics. He receives a call one day from Richard P, a physiologist and researcher at another research university who is a world-renowned expert on hypothermia.

Richard is calling Andrew to ask for ethical advice. He has conducted internal review board approved experiments on cold exposure in human subjects for years in order to develop better ways of dealing with cases of hypothermia. Obvious ethical constraints have stopped him from ever exposing his research subjects to temperatures that might cause lasting harm, but he admits that this has limited some of what he can discover with his research. He is calling Andrew because he knows of experiments conducted in Dachau, the German concentration camp, during World War II on prisoners. Nazi scientists had exposed hundreds of prisoners to freezing temperatures and ice baths to study how humans responded to extreme temperatures. Dozens of prisoners were killed in this research. Richard knows that using Nazi data is controversial. Many ethicists claim that such data are "tainted," and the Environmental Protection Agency once excluded Nazi data from a study on the effects of phosphene gas, asserting that data obtained by such means should never be used in legitimate scientific research. But Richard believes the data collected by Nazi scientists might help in the development of new treatments for hypothermia that have the potential to save many lives. He asks for Andrew's opinion on whether it is ethically defensible to use the Nazi data in his current research.

Questions

1. What are the most significant ethical concerns associated with using Nazi data? How might these concerns be addressed?

2. Should Richard use Nazi data in his research? If not, why? If so, should use of this data be subject to any rules or restrictions?

3. Under what circumstances, if any, would you support use of data that were obtained in ethically questionable experiments?

Resources

Caplan, Arthur L. "How Should We Regard Information Gathered in Nazi Experiments?" *AMA Journal of Ethics* 23, no. 1 (J2021): E55–58. doi: 10.1001/amajethics.2021.55. https://journalofethics.ama-assn.org/article/how-should-we-regard-information-gathered-nazi-experiments/2021-01

Moe, Kristine. "Should the Nazi Research Data be Cited?" *Hastings Center Report* 14, no. 6 (1984): 5–7.

4.2 Research on Prisoners: The Salt Study

Keywords: consent, human subject research, prisoners

Dr. T is part of a research team studying hypertension in American adults. The team is considering the possibility of suggesting a large-scale randomized clinical trial involving 10–20 thousand adults of diverse backgrounds in which participants would be on diets of varied salt-intake levels for five years. The hope is that the data collected in the "Salt Study" could finally answer questions about potential dangers in either high- or low-sodium diets. Although many Americans struggle with hypertension and the American Heart Association has suggested levels of sodium intake for both adults with hypertension and those without, there is a lack of conclusive evidence validating those suggestions. There is even some concern in the medical community that a diet too low in sodium can cause more strokes and heart attacks. Dr. T's research team hopes that with a double-blind, large scale, longitudinal study they will be able to offer evidence-backed suggestions that could improve the lives of many people.

Dr. T and his team argue that the only way to ensure that the diets were strictly followed by participants in the research, however, is to conduct this research on currently incarcerated persons. Prisons are ideal environments for this research because of similarities of lifestyles and the ability to assign a portion of subjects to carefully controlled low-sodium diets while the other subjects continued to receive their normal diet. The team would seek informed consent from the prisoners to participate in the study, though prisoners would not be allowed to determine to which group they would be assigned. There would also be a separate informed consent process for the release of prisoner health data germane to the study to the research group.

The Code of Federal Regulations, which establishes rules for departments and agencies in the federal government, prohibits research on prisoners except in very specific circumstances (45 CFR § 46.306), and biomedical trials are often allowed only when the research impacts the prison population as a particular class or the research has the potential to benefit the individual incarcerated persons participating in the research. Although neither exception applies here, some argue that consensual participation in research that could improve the health of the general population should not be denied to incarcerated persons, especially if the risks are relatively low.

Questions

1. What are the difficulties in obtaining voluntary and informed consent from incarcerated persons? Are these difficulties enough to warrant banning studies like the Salt Study?

2. In what ways, if any, could participation in research like this be considered beneficial for incarcerated persons?

3. The participants in this study would be at relatively low risk of complications given the nature of the study. Would your reasoning change regarding the ethical permissibility of the study if more risk was involved?

4. Should prisoners be compensated for their participation in the study?

Resources

Cornell Law School, Legal Information Institute. "Permitted Research Involving Prisoners." https://www.law.cornell.edu/cfr/text/45/46.306

Kolata, Gina. "The Ideal Subjects for a Salty Study?: Maybe Prisoners." *The New York Times,* June 4, 2018. https://www.nytimes.com/2018/06/04/health/prisoners-salt-study.html?smid=url-share

Maron, Dina Fine. "Should Prisoners Be Used in Medical Experiments?" *Scientific American,* July 2, 2014. https://www.scientificamerican.com/article/should-prisoners-be-used-in-medical-experiments/

4.3 Enrolling a Minor in a Clinical Trial

Keywords: cancer, coercion, consent, human subject research, minors

Johnny B is a 13 year old who has been in treatment for cancer for several years. He has been hospitalized due to multiple complications and, unfortunately, his prognosis is not good. His long-time oncologist, Dr. T, schedules a meeting with Johnny and his family, and includes a new resident physician, Dr. N. Dr. T informs Johnny and his parents that standard treatments for his disease are not working, and he has very limited life expectancy—likely no more than three months. Johnny is tired of struggling with his disease, and he tells the doctor that he hopes they can stabilize him enough to allow him to spend his remaining time at home. But his parents are distraught and reluctant to accept this terrible news. They ask if there is anything else that can be done. Dr. T says that there is a clinical trial being conducted at the hospital and that Johnny can be enrolled. He explains that a new drug has shown promise treating some patients immediately after diagnosis, but it has not proven effective for patients with advanced disease. One of the main goals of the trial is to see how patients like Johnny respond to the drug. Dr. T emphasizes that there is a 50/50 chance Johnny will not be given the new drug but will instead receive an established drug that he has already used without success. The trial will require him to remain in the hospital, undergoing infusions with possible side effects. Above all, Dr. T emphasizes that Johnny and his family should temper their expectations—the best they can hope for is a small extension of Johnny's life expectancy, but it is most likely that he will not realize any significant benefits. The data from the trial will hopefully provide a basis for further research and development, which might help patients like Johnny in the future.

Johnny is not enthusiastic about the trial, particularly because it will require him to stay in the hospital, but his parents are keen to have him participate, seeing it as a better option than simply "giving up." Sensing his parents' distress, Johnny reluctantly agrees to enter the trial.

After they leave the room, Dr. N expresses concern about whether Johnny's wishes and interests are served by enrolling him in the trial. Dr. T responds by saying that medical progress depends on enrolling patients like Johnny in clinical trials; he appreciates Dr. N's concern, but he is satisfied that Johnny is not being coerced. He also notes that Johnny is a minor, and his parents are in charge of his medical decisions.

Questions

1. Dr. N suggests that enrolling Johnny in this trial would deviate from their primary responsibility to promote the interests of their patient. Do you agree?

2. Should physicians pursue therapeutic and research goals with the same patient? If so, how should they balance their responsibilities to patients with their research agenda?

3. What criteria should be considered when determining whether a minor should be enrolled in a clinical trial?

4. What if Johnny strongly objected to entering the trial, but his parents insisted? Would it be ethical for Dr. T to enroll Johnny, based on the fact that his parents are in charge of his medical decisions?

5. Under what circumstances should researchers be prohibited from enrolling minors in clinical trials, even with their parents' permission?

Resource

University of California San Francisco, Human Research Protection Program. "Children and Minors in Research." https://irb.ucsf.edu/children-and-minors-research

4.4 Guinea Pigs: Now Hiring

Keywords: coercion, consent, human subject research

Tyler D is a recent college graduate who is facing a difficult job market. Tyler's roommate, Harry, tells him that he should consider "guinea pigging" as a way to make money until he finds a steady job. When Tyler responds with a puzzled look, Harry explains that "guinea pigging" means being paid by pharmaceutical companies to participate in phase 1 clinical drug trials. He also notes that compensation for volunteers has increased in recent years, as drug companies compete for subjects in their ongoing quest to bring new and more lucrative drugs to market. When Tyler examines websites of pharmaceutical companies that are actively recruiting volunteers, he learns that the compensation is indeed significant. One trial pays up to $12,000 for 6 weeks of services, during which participants must stay at a residence owned by the company and adhere to a restricted diet while they take new drugs and submit to various tests, including bloodwork and endoscopies. The residences are staffed by physicians and researchers, and they offer amenities such as internet service and cable television.

Tyler requests further information about a trial for a rheumatoid arthritis drug in his city, which pays $6,000 for 30 days' work and will require him to stay in a company residence. The company provides information about possible side effects, including damage to his immune system, but assures him that severe side effects are not very likely and that he will be closely monitored by their medical staff. They also inform Tyler that compensation for participants is prorated, with the largest payment provided only on completion of trial. Participants are free to leave at any time, but those who leave before completion only receive a small portion of the final compensation. In addition, Tyler must sign a waiver absolving the company of any liability for injuries he might suffer; if he does suffer illness or side effects from the study, he will be responsible for any needed medical treatment.

This last condition is especially worrisome to Tyler, since he has no health insurance. But he needs money for rent and living expenses, so he decides to enroll in the trial, despite his misgivings.

Questions

1. What ethical concerns arise when drug companies pay volunteers to participate in clinical trials?
2. Should drug companies be allowed to pay human subjects for participation in clinical trials? If so, what rules and regulations should be in place to protect human subjects who are paid to participate?
3. The federal government requires investigators to "minimize the possibility for coercion or undue influence" when they recruit research subjects. Does compensation in this case constitute coercion or undue influence? When would compensation constitute coercion or undue influence?

Resources

Elliot, Carl. *White Coat, Black Hat: Adventures on the Dark Side of Medicine.* Chapter 1: The Guinea Pigs. Boston: Beacon Press, 2010.

PBS.org. *The Poison Squad.* American Experience: Season 32, episode 2, January 28, 2020. ttps://www.pbs.org/wgbh/americanexperience/films/poison-squad/

Walker, Rebecca, L., Marci D. Cottingham, and Jill A. Fisher. "Serial Participation and the Ethics of Health Phase 1 Volunteer Research." *Journal of Medicine and Philosophy* 43, no. 1 (2018): 83–114. https://doi.org/10.1093/jmp/jhx033

World Medical Association. "Declaration of Helsinki: Ethical Principles for Medical Research Involving Human Subjects." https://www.wma.net/policies-post/wma-declaration-of-helsinki-ethical-principles-for-medical-research-involving-human-subjects/

4.5 Vaccine Research for Childhood Diseases in Developing Countries

Keywords: human subject research, minors, vaccines

Researchers involved in an international consortium dedicated to the study of a Common Childhood Virus (CCV) are at a crossroads. The virus they study causes gastroenteritis, an inflammation of the stomach and intestines that causes vomiting and diarrhea. Diarrheal diseases are one of the leading causes of death in children worldwide, specifically in children hailing from low-income nations who are unable to receive adequate treatment for the dehydration and shock that can accompany diarrheal diseases.

An effective vaccine for the virus has been available for almost a decade and is highly effective in preventing virus-induced gastroenteritis. Vaccination against the virus is now part of the vaccine schedule for children in the United States and common in other high-income countries. The World Health Organization has suggested that the addition of this vaccine into the vaccine schedule for infants be a priority in all countries, but especially in countries where access to care for gastroenteritis might be hard to come by.

The researchers in the CCV consortium are torn over an experiment currently being run in the Democratic Republic of Congo (DRC) on a new experimental vaccine for the CCV. Researchers have enrolled 4,000 children in a study. In the study, about one-third of the children enrolled received saltwater injections rather than the vaccine. The new vaccine is heat-stable and does not require refrigeration, unlike the vaccine which has been available for a decade. This has the potential to make distribution of the vaccine in low-income countries much easier, and those conducting the research argue that many thousands of lives will be saved if the vaccine is proven effective. Moreover, they explain, the children in the DRC who receive the saline solution or experimental vaccine would likely not have had access to the established vaccine, so their medical care is not necessarily being worsened by the experiment. Detractors argue that since there is an effective vaccine available, giving some children a placebo is morally reprehensible and disregards established international ethical principles for research on vulnerable human subjects.

Questions

1. Do you think the DRC experiment is justified?
2. Is the DRC experiment consistent with accepted rules governing research on human subjects?
3. If you oppose the experiment, what alternatives might be considered to develop the promising new drug?
4. In your view, what are the most important ethical issues to consider regarding research and experimentation in developing countries?

Resources

Archibong, Belinda and Francis Annan. "What do Pfizer's 1996 Drug Trials in Nigeria Teach Us about Vaccine Hesitancy?" *Brookings.edu.* December 3, 2021. https://www.brookings.edu/blog/africa-in-focus/2021/12/03/what-do-pfizers-1996-drug-trials-in-nigeria-teach-us-about-vaccine-hesitancy/

Rid, Annette, Abha Saxena, Abdhullah H. Baqui, Anant Bhan, Julie Bines, Marie-Charlotte Bouesseau, Arthur Caplan, et al. "Placebo Use in Vaccine Trials: Recommendations of a WHO Expert Panel." *Vaccine* 32, no. 37 (2014): 4708–12. https://doi.org/10.1016/j.vaccine.2014.04.022.

Smith, David. "Pfizer Pays Out to Nigerian Families of Meningitis Drug Trial Victims." *The Guardian,* August 12, 2011. https://www.theguardian.com/world/2011/aug/11/pfizer-nigeria-meningitis-drug-compensation

World Medical Association. "Declaration of Helsinki: Ethical Principles for Medical Research Involving Human Subjects." https://www.wma.net/policies-post/wma-declaration-of-helsinki-ethical-principles-for-medical-research-involving-human-subjects/

4.6 Hacking an Insulin Pump

Keywords: cost of care, health insurance, liability, minors, paternal authority

Jill P is a single mother to 13-year-old Alyssa, who was recently diagnosed with Type 1 diabetes. Although Jill does not have health insurance, Alyssa is covered under a state program for children of families with limited income. Alyssa has been using an insulin pump for a little over five months now, and it's been working well during the day. Alyssa has been good about regularly checking her blood sugar level and adjusting her insulin dosage accordingly. Unfortunately, nights are a mess. Alyssa often experiences blood sugar spikes in the middle of the night, which causes her to wake up often to use the restroom and gives her headaches that can make it hard to fall back asleep. When Jill mentions this to Alyssa's doctor, he tells Jill that there are newer automated insulin delivery systems available that monitor blood sugar levels and dose insulin accordingly, but they are quite expensive. When Jill reaches out to the program that offers Alyssa insurance, she is told that automated insulin delivery systems are not covered.

Jill turns to her online support group for parents of children with diabetes for help. One post she reads talks about "hacking" insulin pumps. Hacking involves linking up the two pieces of technology Alyssa uses to control her diabetes—her insulin pump and her blood glucose monitor—using a smartphone app. The insulin pump and monitor can "talk" with one another in a process called "looping." To do this, Jill would need to source an older, hackable insulin pump and use the online code originally shared by hackers in 2014, OpenAPS. Jill reads several accounts of parents who have set up these "hacked" insulin pumps for their children who were having issues at night just like Alyssa, and learns that this technology has all but eliminated the nighttime glucose spikes. Other patients who have "looped" their devices report a huge improvement in their quality of life now that they don't have to manually monitor blood sugar and adjust their insulin doses in response to everyday activities like eating and exercise.

Jill wonders whether she should consider doing the same for her daughter. Despite the reports of parents who have had success with "hacking" insulin pumps, Jill worries about some of the links posted by other members of the group that warn hacking can be done for nefarious purposes, too, even without a pump's serial number. In fact, the hackable pumps being sold on the secondary market have been recalled by the manufacturer because of security concerns. She also discovers that the FDA has issued a warning stating that looped devices were not designed to be used together, and that looping "could result in inaccurate glucose level readings or unsafe insulin dosing, which can lead to injury requiring medical intervention or death."

These concerns give Jill a pause. She wonders whether looping is the right choice for Alyssa.

Questions

1. Do you think Jill should attempt to hack Alyssa's insulin pump?
2. If you oppose hacking, would your assessment change if Jill was deciding whether to hack her own insulin pump?
3. How should physicians handle conversations with patients who either have hacked pumps or are considering hacking their devices?
4. What steps, if any, should be taken to increase access to FDA-approved monitoring and dosing systems for patients who cannot afford these new products?

Resources

Brown, Dalvin. "Hacking Diabetes: People Break into Insulin Pumps as an Alternative to Delayed Innovation." *USA Today,* June 5, 2019.

US Food and Drug Administration. "FDA Warns People with Diabetes and Healthcare Providers Against the Use of Devices for Diabetes Management Not Authorized for Sale in the United States." May 17, 2019.

https://www.fda.gov/medical-devices/safety-communications/fda-warns-people-diabetes-and-health-care-providers-against-use-devices-diabetes-management-not

Zhang, Sarah. "People Are Clamoring to Buy Old Insulin Pumps." *The Atlantic,* April 29, 2019. https://www.theatlantic.com/science/archive/2019/04/looping-created-insulin-pump-underground-market/588091/

4.7 Direct-to-Consumer Genetic Testing: A Stressful Outcome

Keywords: consent, genetic testing, veracity

Brenda R is an active and healthy 26 year old. She has been seeing Randy W for three years and they are recently engaged. They are both college graduates on promising career paths, Brenda as a medical researcher, and Randy as a civil engineer. They have much to look forward to, and they are planning to buy a house big enough for at least two children. In her workplace, Brenda has heard several coworkers talking about a new genetic sequencing company, KnowYourGenes.com, which touts itself as the most advanced direct-to-consumer genetic information company in the world. In contrast to many companies, KnowYourGenes (KYG) offers a "Platinum" package, which sequences the customer's entire genome. This package costs $500, and includes information about ancestry, health and wellness, and longevity. For an extra fee, the company offers numerous additional reports, including ones that detail the customer's propensity for more than 5,000 diseases, carrier status for genetic diseases, and cognitive and cardio wellness. These reports cost from $40 to $250. The company encourages customers to explore these reports, as part of its mission to provide them with "genetically tailored guidance" and "clear solutions for better health."

Brenda is very curious after exploring the company's website. She purchases the Platinum package and six additional reports, totaling more than $800. When she tells Randy about her purchase, he is very upset. He is concerned that KYG will sell her information, giving other companies access to her personal information. He is especially worried that the reports might affect Brenda's future insurability, by leading companies to exclude coverage for disease propensities or charge higher premiums. He also wonders whether the costly reports will provide Brenda with reliable or actionable information. Randy's concerns escalate when Brenda's reports show that she is at increased risk for several diseases, including early onset dementia and breast cancer, and that she is also a carrier of a rare genetic disorder. Randy expresses his love for Brenda, but says he is very worried about their future—he is especially worried about whether their children will be healthy, and whether he will be able to care for Brenda if she suffers from early onset dementia.

Brenda calls the KYG helpline to express her concerns. The agent tells her that they do not provide information to insurers, but they do provide information to other companies for marketing purposes. They also provide information to law enforcement when needed to assist in criminal investigations, though this is very rare. The agent tells Brenda that her worries about health should be discussed with a genetic counselor. For a $200 fee, the company allows customers to have online discussions with certified genetic counselors for 60 days. Brenda wonders whether she should pay this fee. She wishes she had never purchased the testing, which is causing so much stress in her life.

Questions

1. What can be done to prevent stressful outcomes from genetic testing such as those experienced by Brenda?
2. Should companies be responsible for educating customers about the potential for stressful outcomes of genetic testing? Should they be required to offer genetic counseling?
3. Given the complexity and uncertainty associated with genetic test results, should companies be allowed to claim that these tests provide customers with "genetically tailored guidance" and "clear solutions" to health problems?
4. Should companies be allowed to sell data for marketing purposes if they disclose this to customers in advance?
5. Should law enforcement have access to information gathered in genetic tests? If so, should this access be subject to restrictions?
6. Some countries prohibit direct-to-consumer genetic testing, and only allow doctors to order genetic testing for patients. Would you support such a ban? If so, why? If not, what rules and regulations would you support to govern direct-to-consumer testing companies?

Resources

American College of Obstetricians and Gynecologists. "Committee Opinion No. 410: Ethical Issues in Genetic Testing." June 2008; reaffirmed 2020. https://www.acog.org/clinical/clinical-guidance/committee-opinion/articles/2008/06/ethical-issues-in-genetic-testing

Harris, Anna, Susan E. Kelly, and Sally Wyatt. "Counseling Customers: Emerging Roles for Genetic Counselors in the Direct-to-Consumer Genetic Testing Market." *Journal of Genetic Counseling* 22, no. 2 (2013): 277–88. doi: https://doi.org/10.1007/s10897-012-9548-0

Schaper, Manuel and Silkie Shicktanz. "Medicine, Market, and Communication: Ethical Considerations in regard to Persuasive Communication in Direct-to-Consumer Genetic Testing Services." *BMC Medical Ethics* 19, no. 1 (2018). doi: https://doi.org/10.1186/s12910-018-0292-3

Udesky, Laurie. "The Ethics of Direct-to-Consumer Genetic Testing." *The Lancet* 376 (2010): 1377–78. doi: https://doi.org/10.1016/S0140-6736(10)61939-3

4.8 Making Better Babies

Keywords: eugenics, gene editing

Oscar M is a recent college grad at a prestigious university who double majored in biology and entrepreneurship. He has been talking with some of his fellow grads about a business venture that anticipates new uses of CRISPR (clustered regularly interspaced short palindromic repeats) technology, which allows us to make changes to humans by editing their genes. Oscar is especially interested in gene editing that can be used in conjunction with In Vitro Fertilization, allowing parents to select traits of children at the earliest stage of development. Gene editing is in its infancy, and there are serious concerns about safety and effectiveness, which currently make it ethically problematic. But Oscar and his friends know that science can advance rapidly, and they want to be prepared to take advantage of new opportunities if gene editing becomes safe and effective.

A disagreement has emerged in the group over whether their company should only offer editing to treat diseases, or whether they should also offer editing that allows parents to select for enhancements that would improve their children's chances for happiness and success. Such enhancements could be for physical traits such as height, strength, or appearance; or cognitive traits, such as memory and other attributes associated with intelligence. Several members of the group believe it is immoral to participate in genetic enhancements. They believe this gives parents too much power, and they also express concerns about feeding into a "eugenics mentality." Oscar responds by pointing out that we already allow parents to make important decisions for their children; in fact, we expect good parents to do whatever they can to help make their children's life better. He dismisses the eugenics concern as "dramatic," pointing out that this is the United States, not Nazi Germany. No one is proposing that they try to build a master race! Oscar also emphasizes that genetic enhancement has enormous market potential. If it ever becomes possible to do enhancements safely and effectively, he insists that their company should have a sound marketing plan that will help them get in on the ground level.

Questions

1. What are the most serious ethical arguments against the genetic enhancement of early embryos proposed by Oscar? How might a defender of genetic enhancement respond to these arguments? Do you think genetic enhancement of embryos can be ethically justified?

2. Do the ethical objections to genetic enhancement also apply to gene therapy (i.e., editing that is used to address serious disease)?

3. Would your assessment of genetic enhancement change if it were available only to adults who offer free and informed consent?

4. Do you think companies like the one envisioned by Oscar should be allowed to offer genetic enhancements, provided they can be done safely and effectively? If so, subject to what rules and restrictions?

5. Do you agree that genetic enhancement is a form of "eugenics"? If so, can the same be said of gene therapy, which attempts to eliminate undesirable traits?

Resources

Anderson, W. French. "Genetics and Human Malleability." *Hastings Center Report* 20, no. 1 (1990): 21–24. https://doi.org/10.2307/3562969

Glannon, Walter. "Genetic Enhancement." In Glannon, *Genes and Future People: Philosophical Issues in Human Genetics*, 94–101. Boulder: Westview Press, 2001.

PBS.org. *The Eugenics Crusade*. American Experience: Season 30, episode 9, October 16, 2018. https://www.pbs.org/wgbh/americanexperience/films/eugenics-crusade/

Steinbock, Bonnie. "Designer Babies: Choosing our Children's Genes." *The Lancet* 372 (2008): 1294–95. doi: https://doi.org/10.1016/S0140-6736(08)61538-X

4.9 Deep Brain Stimulation for a Parkinson's Patient

Keywords: consent, depression, neurodegenerative disorder

Marty B is 67 years old, and he has been happily married to Donna for 40 years. Marty was diagnosed with Parkinson's disease just after his 60th birthday, and his symptoms have been worsening despite treatment with a variety of drugs. In addition to severe tremors, he now has difficulty walking and speaking, and he has bouts of fatigue. As his symptoms have worsened, Marty has become severely depressed, and treatment with antidepressants has not proved effective. He is growing despondent, and desperate for anything that might curtail these debilitating symptoms.

Marty and Donna visit Dr. J, a neurologist who specializes in treating Parkinson's. Dr. J suggests Marty might benefit from Deep Brain Stimulation (DBS). This requires implanting electrodes in his brain that are connected to a stimulator that is placed under the skin below his collarbone. The stimulator is programmed to generate electrical impulses that control abnormal activity in his brain. Dr. J notes that DBS has proved to be a highly effective treatment for some Parkinson's patients, and it has also proved effective in treating epilepsy, obsessive compulsive disorder, and depression. He explains that the treatment is not without risks. The surgery to implant electrodes has some risks, including the possibility of bleeding and infection, and the device will need to be adjusted to deal with possible side effects, including impulse control and mood disorders. Marty feels he has run out of options, and his symptoms are becoming intolerable, so he opts for the surgery to implant the DBS device.

Marty handles the surgery well, and he soon experiences a remarkable reduction of symptoms. His motor symptoms virtually disappear, as does his depression. He has renewed energy and is able to resume activities he thought would no longer be possible. But the DBS treatment also comes with some unwelcome changes. Prior to his surgery, Marty was reserved and mild-mannered, often described by his friends as "mellow Marty." But after the DBS, his newfound energy often borders on mania, and he has greatly increased sexual desire that manifests in ways Donna finds inappropriate. Donna is also troubled by newly emerging compulsive behaviors, including online shopping binges and gambling that are depleting their savings. These behaviors are so out of character that Donna feels like she is living with a new person, not her "pre-Parkinson's husband." She feels unprepared for these unwelcome side effects and wonders whether DBS was the right choice. Though Marty is relieved his symptoms have abated, he recognizes his behavior is problematic and he knows it is putting a serious strain on their marriage.

Marty and Donna schedule a visit with Dr. J to solicit his advice and input.

Questions

1. What advice should Dr. J give to Marty? Do you think Marty should consider turning off the stimulator?

2. Do you think Marty's consent to DBS was sufficiently informed and voluntary? If not, what concerns do you have and what could have been done differently to address these concerns?

3. What do you think of Donna's belief that Marty is "no longer himself"? By manipulating the brain, can DBS and brain-computer interface devices undermine the autonomy and identity of patients?

4. Is Marty responsible for the changes in behavior that occur after the start of DBS? Why or why not? Suppose he committed a crime, such as sexual assault. Should the DBS treatment be taken into account in assessing his moral and/or legal culpability?

Resources

Burwell, Saha, Matthew Sample, and Eric Racine. "Ethical Aspects of Brain Computer Interfaces: A Scoping Review." *BMC Medical Ethics* 18 (2017). https://doi.org/10.1186/s12910-017-0220-y

Drew, Liam. "The Ethics of Brain-Computer Interfaces." *Nature* 571 (2019): S19–21. https://www.nature.com/articles/d41586-019-02214-2

Munoz, Katrina A., Kristin Kostick, Clarissa Sanchez, Lavina Kalwani, Laura Torgerson, et al. "Researcher Perspectives on Ethical Considerations in Adaptive Deep Brain Stimulation Trials." *Frontiers in Human Neuroscience* 14 (2020). https://doi.org/10.3389/fnhum.2020.578695

4.10 Using Wearables to Monitor the Health and Wellness of Employees

Keywords: coercion, consent, privacy, surveillance

Vivian P is a recent college graduate who is starting a job at a large medical technology company. She is excited about her new position, in part because her new employer has a reputation for cultivating a positive and supportive workplace culture. As part of the onboarding process, Lily D, a Human Resources officer, encourages Vivian to participate in the company's wellness program, which is very popular among employees. A centerpiece of this program is state-of-the-art health monitoring. Employees who choose to participate are given a smart watch with enhanced monitoring features. The device provides real-time monitoring for a range of vital signs, including pulse, heart rhythm, temperature, and blood oxygen levels. It also monitors sleep and movement patterns and detects changes in vital signs that could be early signs of disease onset. It provides individualized health reports related to cardio-fitness and other health indicators, which employees can access via smartphones and computers, and which they can use to make healthy lifestyle changes. For employees with diagnosed medical problems, the company will provide nanosensors that can be implanted beneath the skin or embedded in a temporary tattoo, which provide more detailed information to help manage their health conditions.

Lily emphasizes that the program is strictly voluntary, but she notes that over 75 percent of the company's employees participate, including her, and she portrays it as a "Win/Win situation." In addition to a smart watch and the benefits of health monitoring, employees who opt in receive a 30 percent reduction in their health insurance premium, as well as free gym membership. The monitoring allows the company to reduce health care premiums for all employees, by providing aggregate information to its insurance carrier about the overall health and wellness of its workers. Moreover, healthy employees tend to be happier and more productive, contributing to the success of the company.

Vivian is intrigued by the wellness program but conflicted about whether to participate. She wants to be a team player who helps contribute to a healthy corporate culture, and she believes the monitoring will help her make some healthy lifestyle changes related to diet and exercise. As a new employee on an entry-level salary, she is especially attracted by the prospect of a free smart watch, a 30 percent premium reduction, and a free membership to a gym right near her apartment. On the other hand, she has some concerns about the privacy of her medical information, and whether it could potentially fall into the wrong hands. But she reasons that 75 percent of her coworkers would not be participating if their privacy was endangered, and she believes her medical information will be protected by HIPPA and other laws. She quickly scans the six-page informed consent form for the program, which Lily assures her is "just a bunch of legalese," and signs on to participate.

Questions

1. Would you participate in this wellness program?
2. Is Vivian's consent to participate in the program sufficiently informed and voluntary?
3. Do you think companies should be allowed to offer employees incentives to participate in wellness programs? Why or why not? What limits, if any, should be placed on the value of the incentives that can be offered?
4. Some key benefits of health monitoring are described in the case. Can you think of potential problems that might arise when employers monitor the health of their employees?
5. What policies and best practices should govern the monitoring of employees' health and wellness? Should these policies and best practices be voluntary or legally mandated?

Resources

Ajunwa, Ifeoma. "Limitless Worker Surveillance." *California Law Review* 105, no. 3 (2017): 735–76. doi: 10.15779/Z38BR8MF94.

Fleming, Hannah-Kaye. "Navigating Workplace Wellness Programs in the Age of Technology and Big Data." *Journal of Science Policy and Governance* 17, no. 1 (2020). https://doi.org/10.38126/JSPG170104

Marchant, Gary E. "What Are Best Practices for Ethical Use of Nanosensors for Worker Surveillance?" *AMA Journal of Ethics* 24, no. 4 (2019): E356–62. doi: 10.1001/amajethics.2019.356

4.11 Physicians Consider Using AI for Diagnosis and Treatment Recommendations

Keywords: artificial intelligence, bias, consent, liability

Dr. L is the chief medical officer at a large metropolitan hospital, and he has called a meeting of medical staff to provide information about a new and potentially revolutionary technology. This technology uses Artificial Intelligence to diagnose and make treatment recommendations by linking medical files of individual patients to large databases of information. Although these technologies are still being developed and studied, initial results are promising, particularly for diagnosis and treatment of certain forms of cancer. Studies have shown that AI diagnostics can identify cancers in radiological images as accurately or, in some cases, more accurately than many physicians. In the not-too-distant future, there is reason to believe AI diagnostics will be superior to humans for diagnosis of some cancers. Dr. L claims that AI diagnostics improve patient outcomes and will also save time by freeing up physicians to treat other patients. He notes that it is already being used extensively in countries like China and Rwanda, and he says the technology will be available in the coming weeks at the hospital. Though use of AI diagnosis will be strictly voluntary, he hopes physicians will take advantage of this opportunity to improve patient care.

When the floor is opened for questions, Dr. Y, a well-respected oncologist, says he is happy to hear that use of the new AI tools will be voluntary. Though he appreciates the potential of these technologies, he says he will stick with "old fashioned" diagnosis and treatment. Dr. Y wonders whether patients will welcome the use of machines rather than humans to diagnose and make treatment recommendations, and he also wonders whether tools developed through use in other countries will be accurate for use on his own patients. In addition, he has serious concerns about liability. What happens if an AI tool misdiagnoses or recommends an ineffective treatment for one of his patient? Would he be liable for this error or would the creator of the algorithm? Dr. Y emphasizes that "no one is perfect," and when things go wrong he would prefer being judged by accepted rules of responsibility and negligence. "If I get sued over a misdiagnosis or treatment, I want to be able to show up in the court to defend myself by explaining why the mistake was made and, hopefully, why it was a reasonable error. If I get sued for an AI mistake, I would have no way to pinpoint and justify the error."

A new physician, Dr. D offers counters by saying that he will almost certainly use the technology when it becomes available. He believes patients expect doctors to use the latest and best technologies, and if AI becomes the best diagnostic tool, he would feel an ethical obligation to use it. In response to Dr. Y's worries about foreign development and applications, Dr. D declares "Cancer is cancer—social differences among patients are not really relevant here." He also questions Dr. Y's concerns about liability, saying "Wait until you make a mistake in an 'old fashioned' diagnosis and get sued by a patient who finds out you decided not to use a more accurate tool provided by the hospital!"

On balance, the medical staff in attendance seem enthusiastic about the new AI technology, despite Dr. Y's concerns.

Questions

1. If AI diagnosis becomes more accurate than human diagnosis, and enables doctors to serve more patients, would doctors have an ethical obligation to use it?

2. If an AI algorithm makes a mistaken diagnosis or treatment recommendation, who should be liable? The doctor, the manufacturer of the AI device, or the medical institution?

3. Should doctors tell patients when they are using AI for purposes of diagnosing or making treatment recommendations? Should patients be able to decide whether they want to be evaluated with AI tools?

4. Do you think there are clinical and/or ethical issues associated with the social contexts in which AI tools are developed and deployed? If so, what are these issues and how might they be addressed?

5. In your view, what are the most significant concerns about diagnosis and recommendation via AI? How might those concerns be addressed?

Resources

Anderson, Michael and Susan Leigh Anderson, "How Should AI Be Developed, Validated, and Implemented in Patient Care?" *AMA Journal of Ethics* 21, no. 2 (2019): E125–30. doi: 10.1001/amajethics.2019.125

Grote, Thomas, and Philip Berens. "On the Ethics of Algorithmic Decision-making in Healthcare." *Journal of Medical Ethics* 46, no. 3 (2020): 205–11. http://dx.doi.org/10.1136/medethics-2019-105586

Kempt, Hendrick and Saskia K. Nagel. "Responsibility, Second Opinions and Peer-Disagreement: Ethical and Epistemological Challenges of Using AI in Clinical Diagnostic Contexts." *Journal of Medical Ethics* 48, no. 4 (2022): 222–29. http://dx.doi.org/10.1136/medethics-2021-107440

Luxton, David D. "Should Watson Be Consulted for a Second Opinion?" *AMA Journal of Ethics* 21, no. 2 (2019): E131–37. doi: 10.1001/amajethics.2019.131.

4.12 Tracking Dementia Patients

Keywords: consent, neurodegenerative disorder, privacy, surveillance

Lydia K is the mayor of a mid-size West Coast city with a reputation for progressive civic policies. The city is notably committed to promoting the health and safety of citizens through creative initiatives, and Lydia is meeting with the City Council to discuss a health concern. In recent months, the city has experienced several tragedies involving elderly dementia patients who were harmed or killed after they wandered from their homes or care facilities and got lost. In response, Lydia proposes a plan that is modeled on one adopted in the Japanese city of Itami, which has also struggled to address concerns about the safety of dementia patients in its aging population. Itami has more than 1,000 sensors throughout the city, which can be used to track dementia patients. Families insert cards in the wallets or clothing of their loved ones, and the sensors detect these cards to show their exact location. This promotes the safety and wellness of dementia patients, and provides peace of mind to their families.

Lydia knows that Americans, even in progressive communities, are wary of government surveillance. But she also knows the citizens are committed to care for the elderly, and she notes that motion monitors and tracking devices for dementia patients are widely marketed and employed in the United States. She thinks her monitoring system is a reasonable and efficient extension of current monitoring practices, which will provide tangible benefits to dementia patients, their families, and the community at large. She also points out that the monitors in Itami are being widely used to track elementary school students as they walk to and from schools, and she believes parents in their city will be enthusiastic about the prospect of this additional application.

Opinions on the council are mixed. Some members support the proposal, but others wonder whether it is right to track sick people as if they are "criminals" and express concerns about creeping toward a "police state." The proposal is tabled pending public input.

Questions

1. What are the most significant ethical issues raised by this tracking technology?
2. Can you think of any unforeseen negative consequences that might result from implementation of this tracking technology?
3. Would you support the use of this monitoring system? If so, what rules and regulations should govern the use of this technology? Should patient consent be required or only consent of families?
4. If available, would you consider using this technology to monitor a member of your family who has dementia?

Resource

Dooley, Ben and Hisako Ueno. "Where a Thousand Digital Eyes Keep Watch over the Elderly." *The New York Times,* February 2, 2022.

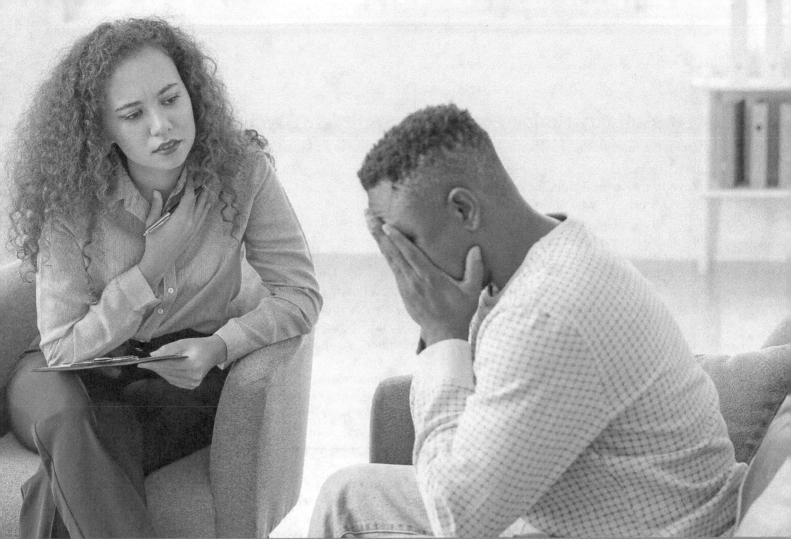

CHAPTER 5

Behavioral and Mental Health

5.1 A Halfway House Patient Discontinues Psychiatric Medication

Keywords: mental illness, nonadherence, resource allocation, veracity

Julie K is a social worker in charge of Hope House, a recovery house for those living with mental illness who were recently released from inpatient treatment. Hope House hosts up to twelve adults at a time and provides a place for persons who are recovering from prolonged periods of severe mental illness, but who no longer qualify for inpatient psychiatric treatment. There is always a long list of patients who are waiting for a bed at Hope House.

One of Hope House's current guests, Sylvia P, has been staying at Hope House for about two weeks. She was previously hospitalized for two months for Bipolar 1 Disorder and has a history of self-harm and cutting. She was hospitalized after attempting suicide following a severe depressive episode. During her two months in hospital, Sylvia was stabilized via a combination of therapy and medication, and after it was determined that she was no longer actively suicidal, she was discharged to Hope House. During her time at Hope House, Sylvia has been compliant with her treatment regimen of medication and intensive outpatient therapy.

Sylvia is seeing Julie for a one-on-one session and Sylvia mentions to Julie that she has stopped taking one of the medications she's been prescribed, quetiapine, an antipsychotic. She says it has made her put on weight and feel groggy. She reports that she just does not feel like herself on the medication. When Julie presses Sylvia on this and explains to her how dependent her recovery is on her compliance with treatment, Sylvia gets agitated and aggressive, and tells Julie that she shouldn't be forced to put anything in her body that she does not want.

Julie knows that medication nonadherence is a frequent problem in those with Bipolar Disorder, but she is also aware of Hope House's policy regarding medication nonadherence: If a guest refuses to follow the regimen prescribed by Hope House's psychiatrist, they need to find alternate living arrangements. Julie feels like she and Sylvia have developed trust and that she might be able to convince Sylvia to continue taking her medication within some time, but Hope House policy dictates that she should record Sylvia's noncompliance in her notes, which are reviewed by the psychiatrist. Julie worries that if the psychiatrist confronts Sylvia, she will refuse the medication and be kicked out of Hope House. Julie knows that there are a large number of patients on the waiting list, and any noncompliance on Sylvia's part will make it seem like she's "taking up a bed" that could be used by a more compliant guest.

Questions

1. Should Julie make a note of Sylvia's nonadherence in her treatment notes?
2. Since a common feature of Bipolar Disorder is medication nonadherence, is it ethical for Hope House policy to require immediate adherence to a medication regimen by those with the disorder?
3. Does the long waiting list of potential guests to Hope House factor into your reasoning about this case?
4. New technology allows for the prescription of "trackable pills." Each pill is equipped with a small sensor and the patient to whom the drugs are prescribed wears a sensor on their chest or stomach, which records the presence of the sensor every time medication is taken. Do you think it is ethical to use trackable pills to monitor medication adherence of psychiatric patients?

Resources

Rahman, Tahir. "Should Trackable Pill Technologies Be Used to Facilitate Adherence Among Patients Without Insight?" *AMA Journal of Ethics* 21, no. 4 (2019): E332–36. https://doi.org/10.1001/amajethics.2019.332.

Srivastava, Shefali. "Ethics Commentary: Bipolar Disorder: Ethical Considerations in the Treatment of Bipolar Disorder." *FOCUS* 9, no. 4 (2011): 461–64. https://doi.org/10.1176/foc.9.4.foc461.

5.2 A Patient Refuses Medication in a Psychiatric Advance Directive

Keywords: advance directive, depression, mental illness, surrogate decision making

Maria J is a 57-year-old woman diagnosed with Bipolar 1 Disorder (BPD). She has a history of manic and depressive episodes since her early 20s and was diagnosed with BPD in her late 20s, when she started taking medications to help manage her BPD. For the first few years Maria did not always follow her medication regime, but she eventually took her medication regularly and developed a long-standing relationship with a psychiatrist. About two years ago, Maria worked with her psychiatrist to taper off one of her medications, an antipsychotic, that was causing her significant side effects, including lipid abnormalities and weight gain. Without this medication, the side effects abated, and she has been functioning well.

In the course of her care, Maria worked with her psychiatrist and husband to create a psychiatric advance directive (PAD), which specifies her preferences in the case of a mental health emergency that prevents her from making her own health care decisions. Her PAD states that she should be treated with antidepressants even against her wishes, but that she should not be given the antipsychotic medication that caused side effects.

A few weeks ago, Maria started showing signs of mania that led her husband to seek involuntary hospitalization. Her husband asks her care team to try to treat Maria without putting her back on antipsychotics. He knows that when Maria is well, she will refuse the medication. After a week in the psychiatric unit at the hospital, Maria is still suffering with symptoms of psychosis. She exhibits paranoid tendencies and hears voices and lashes out at her caregivers. She reports to her care team that aliens are coming to take her away and is often frightened and upset. The care team approaches her husband about putting Maria on a short course of antipsychotic medications to help stabilize her, but he is reluctant to consent.

Questions

1. How should members of Maria's care team advise her husband? What steps should they take if he continues to request Maria not be treated with antipsychotics?
2. What are the key benefits of PADs? What are the most significant challenges associated with PADs?
3. When, if ever, do you think clinicians are justified in overriding PADs? Is overriding a psychiatric advance directive morally different from overriding a standard advance directive?

Resources

Hindley, Guy, Lucy A. Stephenson, Alex Ruck Keene, Larry Rifkin, Tania Gergel, and Gareth S. Owen. "'Why Have I Not Been Told about This?': A Survey of Experiences of and Attitudes to Advance Decision-making amongst People with Bipolar." *Wellcome Open Research* 4, no. 16 (2019): 1–38. https://www.ncbi.nlm.nih.gov/pmc/articles/PMC6492047.2/

National Resource Center on Psychiatric Advance Directives. https://nrc-pad.org/

Swanson, Jeffrey W., S. Van McCrary, Marvin S. Schwartz, Eric B. Elbogen, and Richard A. Van Dorn. "Superseding Psychiatric Advance Directives: Ethical and Legal Considerations. *Journal of the American Academy of Psychiatry and the Law Online* 34, no. 3 (2006): 385–94.

5.3 A Patient Refuses to Be Cleaned

Keywords: capacity, consent, religion

Jen B, an ethicist at a regional behavioral health inpatient facility, receives a call from Dr. F, the admitting doctor on duty. Dr. F explains that a patient, Mercy M, has been sent to them from the local ER, where she was admitted after the police observed her mumbling to herself and running into traffic repeatedly. She was distressed at being brought to the hospital, but she was given medication and stabilized enough to be transported to the behavioral health facility.

Mercy has obviously been living rough and is dirty, refusing to be cleaned, and screams whenever anyone touches her hair. Mercy also has dreadlocks, and when aides were trying to get Mercy into new clothes, they noticed that spiders and other bugs had infested her locs. Dr. F is unsure what to do. It is clear that Mercy needs to be cleaned, but she will need to be sedated to do so. Dr. F also wonders whether it is ethical to shave Mercy's locs. It seems to be the only way to take care of the infestation, but he recognizes that it is also much more invasive and permanent than the sort of cleaning other patients have been subjected to. Dr. F asks Jen whether he should sedate Mercy for cleaning and, if so, whether cleaning should include shaving her head.

Questions

1. Should Mercy be sedated for cleaning? Why or why not? If so, should cleaning include shaving her head?
2. What advice should Jen give to Dr. F?
3. Assume Mercy is under 18, but her guardians are unknown. Would that impact your reasoning on this case?
4. Assume Mercy is black and a practicing Rastafarian. Should considerations of racial justice and religious exemptions factor into the decision whether to shave Mercy's locs?

Resources

Ryan, Christopher James, and Jane Bartels. "Involuntary Hospitalization." In *Psychiatric Ethics,* edited by Sidney Bloch and Stephen A. Green, 279–98. New York: Oxford University Press, 2021. https://doi.org/10.1093/med/9780198839262.003.0012.

Testa, Megan and Sara G. West. "Civil Commitment in the United States." *Psychiatry* 7, no. 10 (2010): 30–40.

5.4 A Homeless Patient Leaves the Hospital against Medical Advice

Keywords: capacity, homelessness, liability, nonadherence

Lisa N, a "frequent flier" at an Emergency Department in an urban hospital, came to the ED again this morning with complaints about a giant pressure ulcer and intense pain in her left foot, in which she has a significant bone infection (osteomyelitis). Lisa was admitted and became agitated while waiting for the doctor to come see her. She decided to leave the hospital without consulting anyone and left in her hospital gown in her wheelchair.

Lisa's long history at the hospital reveals that at times it has been determined that she has capacity to make decisions for herself about her care, but at other times she has lacked that capacity. No capacity determination was made when she was admitted, so no paperwork exists that demonstrates that she lacks capacity today. This is also not the first time she has left the hospital against medical advice. Lisa has also been advised many times that she should have her left foot amputated because of her infection, but she has refused amputation since she is unhoused and does not want to move into a shelter or halfway house. Lisa has no known relatives, nor is it known where she is living.

A member of her care team followed Lisa when she left the hospital. He reports that she is sitting across the street from the hospital on her wheelchair, and while she talks with him, she refuses to come back into the hospital. The care team wonders what to do and evaluates several options that all seem bad.

Questions

1. What options might be available to the team? What should the care team do if Lisa continues to refuse to come back into the hospital? Would it be ethical to not intervene at all?

2. Once a patient leaves the hospital, capacity determinations are no longer in the hands of health care workers and often fall to the police. Would it be ethical for the care team to call the police to evaluate Lisa for a psych hold?

3. Should the fact that Lisa is unhoused factor into the team's reasoning? Why or why not?

Resources

Markusic Wimberly, Jennifer, and John Z. Sadler. "How Bodily Integrity Is a Core Ethical Value in Care of Persons Experiencing Homelessness." *AMA Journal of Ethics* 23, no. 11 (2021): E893–97. https://doi.org/10.1001/amajethics.2021.893.

Salhi, Bisan A., Melissa H. White, Stephen R. Pitts, and David W. Wright. "Homelessness and Emergency Medicine: A Review of the Literature." Edited by Alice M. Mitchell. *Academic Emergency Medicine* 25, no. 5 (2018): 577–93. https://doi.org/10.1111/acem.13358.

Reference

Adapted from Bioethics Bowl Cases 2021. Case 10.
https://drive.google.com/file/d/1vveHh1XlAd-ArxWBnvfjLINhdqIDAWjn/view

5.5 Pain Treatment for an Addict

Keywords: addiction, nursing, pain treatment

Nurse H just started her first job as a nurse in the Emergency Department of a hospital in a major metropolitan area. Even a few months in, she's become familiar with the ED's "frequent fliers"—that is, patients who are in and out of the ED for various reasons, whether it is the treatment of chronic illness or lack of access to other care. One of the ED's frequent fliers, Frank C, is a heroin addict with opioid use disorder (OUD) who appears in the ED every few weeks for some sort of ailment related to his drug use or living rough. Tonight, though, Frank shows up with bruises all over his body and explains he slipped on ice and fell downstairs, complains of intense pain in his left arm, and is more agitated than she's ever seen him. Dr. M, the doctor on duty, orders an X-ray and it's discovered that Frank has a fracture in his left radius that will require surgery. The doctor also prescribes a Ketorolac injection for pain management. Even after the Ketorolac is administered, Frank complains of extreme pain and is unable to lay still. Nurse H knows that in cases similar to this and when a patient is in as much pain as Frank appears to be, opioids are often prescribed. She asks the doctor to consider prescribing something stronger while Frank waits to be operated on. The doctor says that this is a clear example of drug-seeking behavior, and that after some time on the job she will be able to see this too.

Questions

1. Is Dr. M justified in withholding opioid medication from Frank?
2. Is Nurse H right to be concerned about the undertreatment of Frank's pain? How should she proceed if Dr. M continues to refuse to prescribe Frank opioids?
3. What are some of the ethical and clinical challenges associated with treating pain in patients with OUD? What best practices might be used to ensure that all patients, regardless of whether they suffer from OUD, receive adequate pain management?

Resources

Dever, Coleen. "Treating Acute Pain in the Opiate-Dependent Patient." *Journal of Trauma Nursing* 24, no. 5 (2017): 292–99. https://doi.org/10.1097/JTN.0000000000000309.

Faria da Cunha, Brooke. "Ethics and Undertreatment of Pain in Patients with a History of Drug Abuse." *Medsurg Nursing* 24, no. 1, (2015): 4–7, 16.

Paschkis, Zoe and Mertie L. Potter. "Pain Management for Patients with Opioid Use Disorder." *The American Journal of Nursing* 115, no. 9 (2015): 24–32.

5.6 An Affair of the Demented

Keywords: consent, neurodegenerative disorder

Mrs. O and Mr. J are residents at Shady Pines Nursing home. Mrs. O is 73 and is diagnosed as mildly demented. She has been widowed for 10 years. Mr. J is also 73 and diagnosed with mild-to-moderate dementia. He has been widowed for 12 years.

Mrs. O and Mr. J struck up an immediate friendship when Mrs. O moved to Shady Pines six months ago. About two weeks into their friendship, Mrs. O and Mr. J entered into a sexual relationship. The two are rarely seen apart at the facility, and Mr. J frequently wants to spend the night with Mrs. O. While Mrs. O knows that Mr. J is not her husband, it is clear that Mr. J does believe Mrs. O is his deceased wife at times. When the staff has tried to remove Mr. J from Mrs. O's room, Mrs. O becomes agitated and will not settle until Mr. J is allowed to stay with her or until she is medicated.

Mr. J's two children are happy about his relationship with Mrs. O. They report that he seems happier than he has in the two years he has lived at Shady Pines. Mrs. O's daughter, however, is appalled at the relationship and wonders if her mother can actually give consent to engage in a relationship with Mr. J. She says her mother said she was "done with all of that," when asked shortly after her husband died whether she would try to find a romantic partnership again, and that there was no way that Mrs. O would be involved with Mr. J if she wasn't experiencing dementia. The staff at Shady Pines has mixed reactions to the affair. Several caregivers think the relationship is morally inappropriate, and they resent the additional time it takes for them to manage the dynamics of the relationship. They also point out that Mrs. O does not always sleep well when Mr. J spends the night, which exacerbates her symptoms the following day. Other members see no problem with the relationship, and believe it is on balance beneficial to the quality of life of both patients.

Questions

1. Should the care facility allow the relationship between these two patients to continue? If so, how should it be managed?
2. How would you assess Mrs. O's daughter's concern about consent?
3. How should care facilities handle romantic relationships between dementia patients? Should they be allowed? If so, under what conditions?

Resources

Belluck, Pam. "Sex, Dementia and a Husband on Trial at Age 78." *The New York Times*, April 13, 2015. https://www.nytimes.com/2015/04/14/health/sex-dementia-and-a-husband-henry-rayhons-on-trial-at-age-78.html.

Ehrenfeld, Mally, Nili Tabak, Gila Bronner, and Rebecca Bergman. "Ethical Dilemmas Concerning Sexuality of Elderly Patients Suffering from Dementia." *International Journal of Nursing Practice* 3, no. 4 (1997): 255–59. https://doi.org/10.1111/j.1440-172X.1997.tb00110.x.

Metzger, Eran. "Ethics and Intimate Sexual Activity in Long-Term Care." *AMA Journal of Ethics* 19, no. 7 (2017): 640–48. https://doi.org/10.1001/journalofethics.2017.19.7.ecas1-1707.

Tarzia, Laura, Deirdre Fetherstonhaugh, and Michael Bauer. "Dementia, Sexuality and Consent in Residential Aged Care Facilities." *Journal of Medical Ethics* 38, no. 10 (2012): 609–13. https://doi.org/10.1136/medethics-2011-100453.

Reference

Adapted from Parks, Jennifer A. and Victoria S. Wilke. *Bioethics in a Changing World*. 1st edition, 590. New Jersey: Pearson, 2010.

5.7 Covert Administration of Medication to a Nursing Home Resident

Keywords: autonomy, consent, neurodegenerative disorder, veracity

Tony B is an 85-year-old resident of a nursing home. He is at the beginning stages of dementia, and is experiencing sundowning, or late day confusion, sometimes dealt with by dementia patients. Most of the time, however, Tony is lucid and seems like himself. One of his medications must be administered around dinner time, the time that Tony often is confused and anxious. The nursing assistants are having a hard time getting Tony to take this medication; he fights with the assistants and accuses them of trying to harm him. The attempts to get Tony to take his medication end up leaving him stressed and upset, and he often has trouble settling down after dinner. The nightly episodes are also stressful for staff members and other patients.

When Tony's daughter, Amanda, comes to visit, Tony's doctor mentions the issue to her and explains that they're considering administering the medication crushed up in Tony's nightly pudding. Amanda is disturbed by this and tells the doctor not to treat her father like a child. The doctor knows that Amanda has only seen her father during the day and has yet to witness one of his sundowning episodes. He also knows that Tony's quality of life is being adversely affected by the nightly struggles over his medication.

Questions

1. Should the doctor authorize covert administration of medication for Tony? Why or why not? Would doing so violate Tony's autonomy?

2. Under what circumstances, if any, should nursing homes administer medications covertly to residents? What guidelines should be followed when medications are administered covertly?

Resources

Abdool, Rosalind. "Deception in Caregiving: Unpacking Several Ethical Considerations in Covert Medication." *Journal of Law, Medicine and Ethics* 45, no. 2 (2017): 193–203.

Lin, Matthew. "Who Should Implement Force When It Is Needed and How Should It Be Done Compassionately?" *AMA Journal of Ethics* 23, no. 4 (2020): E311–17. https://journalofethics. ama-assn.org/article/who-should-implement-force-when-its-needed-and-how-should-it-be-done-compassionately/2021-04

Munden, L. Martina. "The Covert Administration of Medications: Legal and Ethical Complexities for Health Care Professionals." *Journal of Law, Medicine and Ethics* 45, no. 2 (2017): 182–92.

Simpson, Christy. "Covering It Up? Questions of Safety, Stigmatization, and Fairness in Covert Medication Administration." *Journal of Law, Medicine and Ethics* 45, no. 2 (2017): 204–11.

5.8 Following a Patient's Social Media Use

Keywords: mental illness, nonadherence, privacy

Dr. Z is a psychiatrist specializing in mood disorders in adolescents. She has been seeing Jenna B, a 19 year old diagnosed with Bipolar 1 Disorder for almost three years. Jenna has required hospitalization after experiencing a manic episode with psychotic symptoms and it was during that hospitalization when she became a patient of Dr. Z. Before her hospitalization, Jenna had experienced a manic episode during which she stopped taking the medications her first provider had prescribed. In the three years Dr. Z has treated Jenna, her mania has mostly been under control, though she has struggled with severe depressive episodes recently and Dr. Z has been adjusting Jenna's medications to try to get these under control.

In her appointment with Jenna today, Dr. Z notices that Jenna is having trouble sitting still and that when she expresses herself, she is not as clear or coherent as normal. Dr. Z asks Jenna if she has noticed this about herself, and Jenna responds that she is just excited about starting college in the fall and a social media account she just started that allows users to share short videos they create. Jenna explains that she thinks she has the chance to attract a large following on this platform, given that she is "discussing topics of great import to the world" and is attempting to "elevate the consciousness" of her viewers. Dr. Z asks if Jenna is taking her medications as prescribed, and Jenna is less than forthcoming, but eventually responds with "of course." All day after Jenna's appointment, Dr. Z worries about the possibility that Jenna has ceased taking her medications and wonders whether it is appropriate to look her up on the social media platform Jenna mentioned in order to see the content of her videos to look for signs of an oncoming manic episode.

Questions

1. Would it be appropriate for Dr. Z to check Jenna's social media account to see if there is evidence that she is not taking her medications? Why or why not?

2. If Jenna's social media posts indicate that she is not taking her medication or is suffering from uncontrolled symptoms, how should Dr. Z respond?

3. Under what circumstances, if any, do you think it is appropriate for a doctor to examine social media for information that might be relevant to a patient's treatment?

Resources

DiLillo, David and Emily B. Gale. "To Google or Not to Google: Graduate Students' Use of the Internet to Access Personal Information about Clients." *Training and Education in Professional Psychology* 5, no. 3 (2011): 160–66. https://doi.org/10.1037/a0024441.

Jent, Jason F., Cyd K. Eaton, Melissa T. Merrick, Nicole E. Englebert, Susan K. Dandes, Ana V. Chapman, and Eugene R. Hershorin. "The Decision to Access Patient Information From a Social Media Site: What Would You Do?" *Journal of Adolescent Health* 49, no. 4 (2011): 414–20. https://doi.org/10.1016/j.jadohealth.2011.02.004.

Wu, Katherine S. and Janet L. Sonne. "Therapist Boundary Crossings in the Digital Age: Psychologists' Practice Frequencies and Perceptions of Ethicality." *Professional Psychology: Research and Practice* 52, no. 5 (2021): 419–28. https://doi.org/10.1037/pro0000406.

5.9 Force Feeding an Anorexic Patient

Keywords: autonomy, capacity, coercion, difficult patient, mental illness

Beatrice L is a 21-year-old woman who has been hospitalized eight times over the past seven years for anorexia nervosa. She lives with her parents, who bring her to the hospital again after they find her passed out in her bathroom. Beatrice woke up on the way to the hospital and demanded her parents to take her home, but was too weak to act on her wishes. Examination at the hospital reveals that she has a BMI of 13, is hypotensive, and is cachectic.

Beatrice has participated in many modalities of therapy over the years, in addition to her hospitalizations. In addition to outpatient psychodynamic and behavioral therapy, Beatrice was a patient for 6 months at a specialized eating disorder inpatient program when she was first diagnosed with anorexia nervosa at 14. Her parents admitted her to that program against her will, but she made significant physical progress in the time she was there and was released from the program with a BMI of 18.

Soon after being released from the inpatient program, however, Beatrice began to severely restrict her eating again, sometimes eating as few as 200 calories a day. She's become known at the hospital as a difficult patient. When she's been admitted in the past, she refuses to eat, has needed to have a nasogastric (NG) tube inserted for refeeding, and has pulled out the NG tube if not physically or chemically restrained. She's often verbally abusive and aggressive toward the nurses and doctors who treat her.

Beatrice is admitted to the hospital despite her demands to be allowed to go home. She tells her team and parents that she does not want an NG tube under any circumstances. Her parents ask that refeeding Beatrice should begin immediately and suggest inserting the NG tube after anesthetizing Beatrice. They explain how violent and agitated Beatrice has been in the past during insertion and want to avoid traumatizing her in that way. Beatrice's doctor, Dr. F, agrees that the NG tube is necessary to save Beatrice's life, but wonders whether her waking up with an NG tube after being anesthetized would be more traumatic on Beatrice than simply being sedated during insertion and would destroy any trust Beatrice might have for her treatment team.

Questions

1. Does Beatrice have the capacity to consent or refuse the treatment?
2. Should Dr. F cede to Beatrice's parents' request and anesthetize her before inserting the NG tube?
3. Are there cases in which the force feeding of an anorexic patient might not be justified, even if the patient will die without intervention? If so, what would distinguish these cases?

Resources

Jorgensen, Sarah. "Woman with Severe Eating Disorder Wins Right to Refuse Forced Feedings." *CNN*, November 23, 2016. https://www.cnn.com/2016/11/23/health/nj-woman-eating-disorder-legal-case/index.html.

Lavoie, Melissa and Angela S. Guarda. "How Should Compassion Be Expressed as a Primary Clinical and Ethical Value in Anorexia Nervosa Intervention?" *AMA Journal of Ethics* 23, no. 4 (2021): 298–304. https://doi.org/10.1001/amajethics.2021.298.

5.10 DNR for a Previously Suicidal Patient

Keywords: advance directive, code status, mental illness, suicide

Dr. R has owned a thriving psychiatry practice for two decades. She has treated Deb T, a 61-year-old woman, diagnosed with Bipolar Disorder and borderline personality disorder for 16 of those 20 years. Deb has lived a hard life. She has experienced physical, sexual, and psychological abuse in her family of origin, and has been suicidal since she was 15. Deb has attempted suicide no fewer than 10 times since then and has been hospitalized after seven of the attempts, and while medications and therapy have sometimes helped reduce her suicidal thoughts and behaviors, they have never really abated entirely. Her last suicide attempt was over two years ago.

In addition to her mental health diagnoses, Deb also suffers from a number of physical ailments, including chronic obstructive pulmonary disorder, diabetes, migraines, and edema that make it hard for her to walk further than to her mailbox at the end of her short driveway. Her physical health is poor, and she is often hospitalized with respiratory disorders. She's almost died twice from pneumonia.

Deb comes to an appointment with Dr. R one day with her adult sister Peggy, who helps care for her. Deb and Peggy want to talk to Dr. R about the possibility of completing a Psychiatric Advance Directive for Deb, which would affirm a Do-Not-Resuscitate order (DNR) and Physician Orders for Life Sustaining Treatment (POLST) that have already been filled out that specify Deb will only receive comfort care the next time she's hospitalized. Deb's primary care physician and pulmonologist have been consulted and agreed to follow the orders. Deb tells Dr. R that she is tired of the hospitalizations, and though she is not actively suicidal, she does not want to ever be ventilated again.

Questions

1. Should Dr. R sign off on a DNR order for Deb? How should Deb's mental health history, including her previous suicide attempts, factor into Dr. R's consideration of Deb's request for a DNR order?

2. If Deb's last suicide attempt had been two months ago rather than two years ago, would your reasoning about this case change?

Resources

Brody, Benjamin. "Who Has Capacity?" *New England Journal of Medicine* 361, no. 3 (2009): 232–33. https://doi.org/10.1056/NEJMp0902230.

Brody, Benjamin D., Ellen C. Meltzer, and Diana Feldman. "Assessing Decision Making Capacity for Do Not Resuscitate Requests in Depressed Patients: How to Apply the 'Communication' and 'Appreciation' Criteria." *HealthCare Ethics Committee Forum* 29, no. 4 (2017): 303–11. https://search-ebscohost-com.gonzaga.idm.oclc.org/login.aspx?direct=true&db=phl&AN=PHL2362504&site=ehost-live&scope=site.

Cook, Renee, Philip Pan, Ross Silverman, and Stephen M. Soltys. "Do-Not-Resuscitate Orders in Suicidal Patients: Clinical, Ethical, and Legal Dilemmas." *Psychosomatics* 51, no. 4 (2010): 277–82.

5.11 Boarding Psychiatric Patients on the Emergency Department

Keywords: mental illness, resource allocation, violence against health care workers

Dr. F is a new intern in an Emergency Department at a teaching hospital in a mid-sized city in the United States. He is learning a lot from his experience in the ED and his attending physician, Dr. P, is open to questions and provides good mentorship.

About two weeks into his ED rotation, Dr. F encounters Freddie T, a 19 year old who has been brought into the ED by police who found him running into traffic. It is clear that Freddie is in the middle of a psychotic episode. He is experiencing extreme agitation, is unable to sit still, and is scratching himself so aggressively that he is drawing blood in places. He explains to Dr. F that he's sure "avenging angels" are coming after him and will kill him. When Dr. F tries to get Freddie to sit down so he can examine him, Freddie lashes out and yells at Dr. F, who jumps back, unsure how to proceed. This is Dr. F's first experience with a psychotic patient, and Dr. P steps in to provide assistance. After sedating Freddie and having him restrained to prevent him from scratching himself, Dr. P turns to Dr. F.

"We will call up to psych and see if they have a spot for Freddie, but they won't," says Dr. P. "And I doubt Meadows, the private psych facility in town, will take him without insurance."

"What about the state psychiatric facility?" Dr. F asks.

"We haven't been able to get a patient in there in months. Funding was cut, they've had staffing shortages, and they're operating at only 50-percent capacity."

"So, what do we do?"

"We'll give Freddie meds for the agitation now and when a psych consult is available we'll treat his psychosis. We will hold him here until he's no longer actively psychotic. Hopefully a bed will open up somewhere in the meantime, but I wouldn't count on it," Dr. P says, shaking his head. "We often have a handful of psych patients stuck in the ED. We know it's not best practice and that boarding psych patients comes with risks for both them and staff, but there's not much else to be done."

Dr. F is concerned. The ED is a chaotic place and it is already clear that Freddie's agitation was not made better by the chaos. Dr. F also realizes that Freddie needs longer-term care than can be provided in the ED to develop a medication and treatment regimen that can help control the underlying mental illness causing his psychosis.

Questions

1. Psychiatric boarding in emergency departments has become a frequent occurrence. What are some of the potential risks to patients?
2. How might psychiatric boarding impact the health care workers who work in emergency departments?
3. What aspects of the U.S. medical system are contributing to the problems described in this case? What steps can hospitals and other health care facilities take to address this problem? What options are available to address systemic issues?

Resources

Nordstrom, Kimberly, Jon Berlin, Sara Nash, Sejal Shah, Naomi Schmelzer, and Linda Worley. "Boarding of Mentally Ill Patients in Emergency Departments: American Psychiatric Association Resource Document." *Western Journal of Emergency Medicine* 20, no. 5 (2019): 690–95. https://doi.org/10.5811/westjem.2019.6.42422.

Simon, Jeremy, Chadd Kraus, Jesse Basford, Elizabeth Clayborne, Nicholas Kluesner, and Kelly Bookman. "The Impact of Boarding Psychiatric Patients on the Emergency Department: Scope, Impact and Proposed Solutions." *American College of Emergency Physicians* (2019). https://www.acep.org/globalassets/new-pdfs/information-and-resource-papers/the-impact-of-psychiatric-boarders-on-the-emergency-department.pdf

5.12 A Political Duty to Warn?

Keywords: duty to warn, mental illness

In 2017 at a psychiatry conference at Yale's School of Medicine, a group of mental health professionals spoke out about what they perceived as a great threat to the safety and security of the United States: then current President Trump's psychological state. Dr. John Gartner, a founding member of "Duty to Warn," a group constituted by mental health professionals who felt Mr. Trump was mentally unfit to be the president, said at the conference that mental health professionals had an ethical duty to inform the American public of the threat Mr. Trump posed to the nation. Dr. Gartner had started an online petition earlier in the year calling for Mr. Trump to be removed from office on the basis of psychological incapacity.

Dr. Gartner, and those who joined him in trying to draw attention to what they considered the threat of Mr. Trump's presidency, justified their speaking out based on what is called the "duty to warn," a legal concept that indicates a health care practitioner can be held legally responsible if they do not warn relevant parties (who are not their patients) of serious threats of harm that they discover in conversations with their patients.

Their position is controversial, however, because of another rule that appears in Section 7 in the American Psychiatric Association's (APA) Principles of Medical Ethics called the Goldwater Rule. This rule requires that psychiatrists refrain from commenting on political candidates' and public figures' mental fitness without personally examining them. This rule was named after 1964 Republican presidential nominee, Barry Goldwater, who was declared unfit for the office of president by over 1,000 psychiatrists in a petition published in *Fact* magazine. Goldwater sued for libel and won. This precedent has made many psychiatrists hesitant to offer professional advice and opinions when requested by journalists or others with concerns about the mental fitness of those in the public eye.

Questions

1. What are the most significant ethical issues raised by the advocacy of the "Duty to Warn" group?
2. What are the strongest arguments in defense of the Goldwater rule for psychiatrists? Is this rule in conflict with a health care worker's legal duty to warn third parties who might be endangered by patients?
3. Should the Goldwater rule be abandoned or revised? If revised, what changes should be made to it?
4. Should health care workers use their professional expertise in nonmedical settings, such as legal proceedings, law enforcement activities, and political campaigns?

Resources

Andrade, G. and M. Campo-Redondo. "The Ethics of Psychiatrists' Political Involvement: A Reassessment in the Trump Era." *Ethics, Medicine and Public Health* 15 (2020): 100554. https://doi.org/10.1016/j.jemep.2020.100554.

Centers for Disease Control and Prevention. "Duty to Warn." May 3, 2021. https://www.cdc.gov/std/treatment/duty-to-warn.htm.

Glass, Leonard L. "The Goldwater Rule Is Broken. Here's How to Fix It." STAT (blog), June 28, 2018. https://www.statnews.com/2018/06/28/goldwater-rule-broken-psychiatrists/.

Sheehy, Gail. "Yale Psychiatrists Cite 'Duty to Warn' About Unfit President." *The Intelligencer*, April 23, 2017. https://nymag.com/intelligencer/2017/04/yale-psychiatrists-cite-duty-to-warn-about-unfit-president.html.

5.13 Telehealth Across State Lines

Keywords: depression, LGBTQ+ issues, mental illness, telemedicine, veracity

Megan E is a licensed clinical social worker with a thriving private counseling practice. She lives in a mid-sized city in a very conservative state, and most of her work is with people who are part of the LGBTQ+ community. She is one of the few practitioners in her region who specialize in LGBTQ+ issues and one of the few practitioners who openly identifies as queer. In order to be as accommodating as possible, she charges patients on a sliding scale and offers teletherapy as an option for those who are unable to travel to meet with her in person.

Megan has been treating Sasha R, a 21-year-old trans woman since before Sasha started transitioning two years ago. Before she began working with Megan three years ago, Sasha was having suicidal thoughts frequently and dealt with major depressive episodes. With therapy and medication, Sasha is doing well. Although she still struggles with depression, her suicidal thoughts have almost completely abated. Making the choice to transition helped a lot.

Sasha is a college student in the town where Megan practices, and her hometown is a few states west. Sasha's family of origin does not know that Sasha is transitioning and would not be supportive. In fact, Sasha worries that they would disown her if they found out. When she visits home, Sasha presents as masculine and uses her deadname. Although it causes her distress to do this, she feels there is no other way to be around her family.

It's the summer before Sasha's senior year and her summer housing in town has fallen through. Sasha tells Megan that she needs to live at home for the summer and is obviously distressed by the idea. Sasha is spinning out about needing to buy masculine clothes, needing to find somewhere to store the contents of her very feminine clothing and decor that she feels she can't bring home, and generally needing to pretend for three months to be someone who she isn't. She asks whether Megan can continue to see her online when she's at home. Megan wants to see Sasha over the summer, but she is not licensed in the state Sasha's family is in. She considers treating Sasha anyway and leaving Sasha's location out of her patient notes. Megan knows that she could lose her license if this is discovered, but she worries what might happen to Sasha if she does not have support.

Questions

1. Should Megan continue to treat Sasha over the summer? If not, what steps might she take to support Sasha?
2. In response to the COVID-19 pandemic, many states made emergency exceptions to allow practitioners who are licensed in other states to provide telehealth services. Should these exceptions be extended now that states have opened back up?
3. Besides licensure requirements, what barriers impede the delivery of telehealth services? How might these barriers be addressed?
4. What are the most significant benefits of telehealth for the delivery of mental health care services? What are the most significant potential risks?

Resources

Appleby, Julie. "Telehealth's Limits: Battle over State Lines and Licensing Threatens Patient's Options." *Kaiser Health News*, August 31, 2021. https://khn.org/news/article/state-medical-licensing-rules-threatens-telehealth-patient-options/

Turner Lee, Nicole, Jack Karsten, and Jordan Roberts. "Removing Regulatory Barriers to Telehealth before and after Covid." *Brookings.edu*, May 6, 2020. https://www.brookings.edu/research/removing-regulatory-barriers-to-telehealth-before-and-after-covid-19/

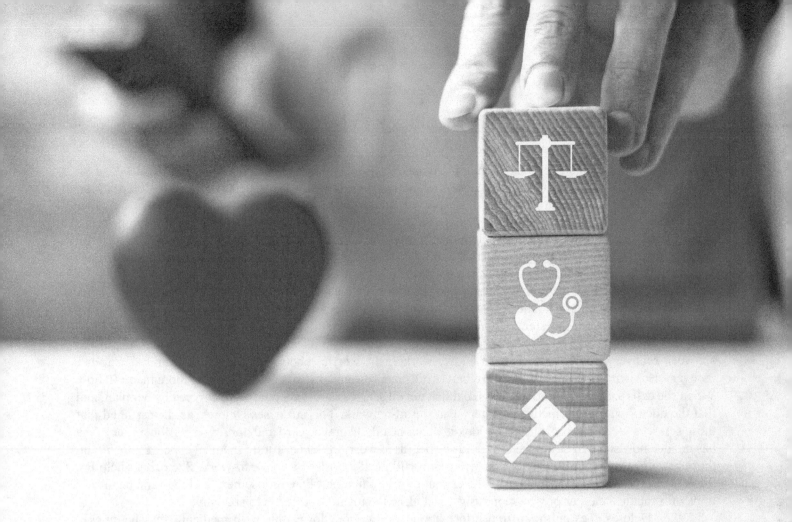

CHAPTER 6

Social Justice and Access to Health Care

6.1 An Insured Worker Struggles with Medical Expenses

Keywords: cost of care, health insurance

Delores G is 34 years old and is just managing to make ends meet. She has been working in the warehouse for a major retailer since graduating high school, and her hourly salary now translates to about $36,000 per year. The job includes health insurance, which is especially important to Delores, since she has diabetes and other health issues that require prescription drugs and occasional doctor's visits. Even with her insurance, she typically pays several thousand per year in deductibles and coinsurance, which she sometimes has to put on credit cards. Although she budgets carefully and works hard to pay down her credit cards, she has accumulated debt of more than $5,000 at high interest.

Delores's challenges are compounded when she is hospitalized with persistent and worsening sores on her right foot, a complication from her diabetes. The wounds are infected and showing loss of tissue, and doctors tell her that this is a life-threatening condition, which can only be effectively addressed through amputation. Delores consents to the surgery, which is performed without complication, and is sent home to begin her six-week recovery. Since Delores is an hourly worker, she worries about keeping up with bills during her recovery. Her worries escalate when she receives bills from the hospital and her surgeon for more than $50,000. When she calls for an explanation, she is told that not all services at the hospital were covered by her plan, and that the doctor who performed her surgery was out-of-network. This surprises Delores, as she assumed that these services were covered when they looked at her health insurance card and approved her for surgery. She has no idea how she will pay these bills, and she begins to worry about her future medical expenses, including those associated with a prosthetic foot, which she will need in order to return to work. She cannot help but think about the worst-case scenario: if she cannot return to her job, she will lose her insurance and be unable to pay for medical care or prescription drugs, including the insulin she needs to stay alive.

When Delores goes online to find information about options for people with medical debt, she quickly encounters numerous stories of people like herself, who are struggling with medical expenses despite having jobs and health insurance. She also learns that nearly 80 million Americans report problems associated with medical expenses and debt, while citizens of other developed countries rarely face these difficulties. She wonders why the United States is willing to allow so many of its citizens to be burdened by medical debt and the stresses that go along with it.

Questions

1. What aspects of our health care system are contributing to Delores's medical expenses? What options are available to Delores for managing her medical debt and securing continued access to health care?

2. Why do so many U.S. citizens experience hardship associated with medical expenses, in comparison to citizens in other countries? What steps might be taken to help reduce this hardship?

3. Some would argue that personal medical debt in the United States is part of the price we pay for our commitment to the free market and for having the best health care in the world. Do you agree with these claims?

4. Should U.S. citizens, like citizens in other developed countries, have access to basic medical care, regardless of their ability to pay? If not, why? If so, how would you define "basic."

5. Countries employ many different models for delivering and paying for medical care. What are the advantages and disadvantages of these models? If you were building a health care system, what features would it include?

Resources

Levy, Noam. "Americans' Struggle with Medical Bills Are a Foreign Concept in Other Countries." *Los Angeles Times*, September 12, 2019. https://www.latimes.com/politics/story/2019-09-11/american-struggle-insurance-deductibles-unique

Levy, Noam and Aneri Pattani. "Medical Debt Upended Their Lives: Here's What It Took from Them." Health News from NPR, June 16, 2022. https://www.npr.org/sections/health-shots/2022/06/16/1104969627/medical-debt-upended-their-lives-heres-what-it-took-from-them

Reid, T.R. *The Healing of America: A Global Quest for Better, Cheaper, and Fairer Health Care.* New York: Penguin Random House Books, 2010.

Scott, Dylan, Ezra Klein, and Tara Golshan. "Everybody Covered: What the US Can Learn from Other Countries' Health Systems." *Vox*, January 13, 2020. https://www.vox.com/2020/1/13/21055327/everybody-covered

6.2 A Patient Faces Impediments to Medications and Health Care

Keywords: cost of care, social determinants of health

Alejandro J is an uninsured 85-year-old man with limited English-language proficiency who has a history of Type 2 diabetes, hypertension, obesity, and nonadherence to medications. Alejandro is a patient at a federally qualified health center (FQHC), and he has been referred by his physician to a bilingual pharmacist, Melinda L, to assist him in managing his chronic medical conditions. Melinda practices in the FQHC clinic as part of an interprofessional team that consists of physicians, nurse practitioners, physician assistants, medical assistants, and dietitians. Melinda works under a collaborative practice agreement (CPA) with the physician, which allows her an expanded scope of practice to initiate, modify, and discontinue medication therapy under the terms of the agreement. During Alejandro's visit, Melinda reviews his chart in the electronic health record. Melinda notices that Alejandro's most recent A1C—a measure of a patient's average blood sugar levels over three months—is 11 percent, indicating that his current medications are either not being taken or, if being taken, are not controlling his diabetes. Melinda also notices that Alejandro has more than one angiotensin-converting-enzyme (ACE) inhibitor prescription. Duplicate use of ACE inhibitors occurs in about 5 percent of elderly patients and often suggests poor communication among clinicians managing a patient's prescriptions. Alejandro also informs Melinda that he had been underdosing his insulin to try to make his supply last longer and admits that he missed a recommended dental appointment because he is saving money for food and bus fare. He inquires how much his new prescriptions will cost.

Questions

1. What social determinants are affecting Alejandro's health care? What steps should Melinda take to try to address these factors?

2. Suppose Melinda worked for a pharmacy that did not participate in the FQHC clinic. What steps, if any, would she be obligated to take to help Alejandro?

3. Should national pharmacy chains be required to have a certain number of pharmacists and locations that participate in FQHC clinics? If so, should this participation be subsidized or incentivized?

4. Can you think of initiatives, community-based or federal, that might help address the needs of patients whose health is impacted by social determinants?

Resource

Shahdoost, Sara Moghadam, and Sandra Leal. "How Should Physicians and Pharmacists Collaborate to Motivate Health Equity in Underserved Communities?" *AMA Journal of Ethics* 23 (2021): E117–26. https://journalofethics.ama-assn.org/article/how-should-physicians-and-pharmacists-collaborate-motivate-health-equity-underserved-communities/2021-02

Reference

From Shahdoost, Sara, Moghadam and Sandra Leal. "How Should Physicians and Pharmacists Collaborate to Motivate Health Equity in Underserved Communities?" *AMA Journal of Ethics* 23 (2021): E117–26. https://journalofethics.ama-assn.org/article/how-should-physicians-and-pharmacists-collaborate-motivate-health-equity-underserved-communities/2021-02

6.3 Rationing Insulin: A Dangerous Decision

Keywords: cost of care, health insurance, social determinants of health

Manny T is 26 years old, and he suffers from Type 1 diabetes. His diabetes has been effectively controlled through insulin, which he must inject several times a day. Manny got a late start in college, deciding to work for a few years at a restaurant after high school to get a sense of independence and to take some of the financial burden off his mom, Julia, who has been a single mom since Manny's father died when he was 10. At age 22, Manny began college at a state school two hours from home, financing his studies with a combination of student loans and a part-time job as a barista. He recently graduated with a degree in biology and began interviewing for entry-level positions in field biology. Unfortunately, it is taking longer than he hoped to land his first "real job." But he has been promoted to manager at the coffee shop, so at least he is able to pay his bills while he continues his job search.

The problem is that Manny is approaching his 27th birthday, which means he will no longer be eligible for coverage under Julia's health insurance plan. His job at the coffee shop does not include health insurance and does not pay enough to cover his insulin and diabetes supplies, which cost nearly $1,400 per month. If he was on Medicaid, his insulin would be paid for, but he makes more than the $18,700 limit for eligibility. He contemplates cutting back his hours to go below this limit, but he discovers that his state did not opt-in for Medicaid expansion under the Affordable Care Act, which means single persons without children are ineligible regardless of income level. He considers buying his own health insurance, but this would cost $400 per month, and he would have to pay $7,900 in drug and medical expenses before the plan would cover his insulin, so he decides this is not financially feasible either. He briefly contemplates going to Canada, where he can acquire his monthly insulin and supplies for more than $1,000 less than in the United States, but he does not have a car and he is not sure he can find a friend to drive him on the 700-mile round trip.

He talks by phone with his mother to discuss possible solutions. Julia urges him to move back home, so he can save money on bills and return to his old job at the restaurant, which would allow him to buy health insurance and cover his deductible while continuing his job search. But Manny values his independence and worries about being a burden to his mother. He tells her he will work extra hard on new job applications and expresses confidence that he will soon be able to find a job with health insurance. In the meantime, he starts rationing his insulin, by lowering his doses or taking shots less frequently, in order to stretch his remaining supply. Less than a week later, Manny experiences severe nausea and weakness at work, and he is rushed to the hospital by a coworker. He is diagnosed with diabetic ketoacidosis and nearly lapses into a coma. He is treated for five days in the hospital before he is well enough to go home.

While recuperating, Manny learns that one in four diabetics in the United States has rationed insulin, and he reads accounts of numerous young people who have died as a result of insulin rationing. He feels lucky to be alive, but he is still worried about how he will pay for his next supply of insulin, not to mention the hefty bill he expects from his hospital stay. The joy of his recent graduation is now overshadowed by concern about his future.

Questions

1. What aspects of the U.S. health care system are making it difficult for Manny to access affordable insulin? What steps might be taken to make insulin more affordable and accessible for patients like Manny?
2. Insulin costs much more in the United States than in Canada and many European countries (about 6 to 12 times more in 2022). Why is insulin so much more expensive in the United States? Is this cost disparity justified? If so, why? If not, what changes might be made to address this disparity?
3. Higher drug prices in the United States are often justified by appeals to the free market, as well as research and development costs. What is your assessment of these justifications?
4. Should drugs like insulin be available to all U.S. citizens regardless of their ability to pay?
5. What are the costs and consequences for a society when citizens cannot access prescription drugs and medical care, or can only do so at great financial hardship?

Resources

Cefalu, William T., Daniel E. Dawes, Gina Gavlak, Dana Goldman, William H. Herman, Karen Van Nuys, Alvin C. Powers, et al. "Insulin Access and Affordability Working Group: Conclusions and Recommendations" *Diabetes Care* 41 (2018): 1299–1311. https://doi.org/10.2337/dci18-0019

Human Rights Watch. "If I'm Out of Insulin, I'm Going to Die: United States' Lack of Regulation Fuels Crisis of Affordable Insulin." April 12, 2022. https://www.hrw.org/report/2022/04/12/if-im-out-insulin-im-going-die/united-states-lack-regulation-fuels-crisis

Sable-Smith, Bram. "Insulin's High Cost Leads to Lethal Rationing." Health News from NPR, September 1, 2018. https://www.npr.org/sections/health-shots/2018/09/01/641615877/insulins-high-cost-leads-to-lethal-rationing

6.4 Relinquishing Child Custody to Obtain Mental Health Treatment

Keywords: cost of care, health insurance, mental illness

Linda, 47, is a single mother to 16-year-old Tommy. Tommy has experienced behavioral and mental health issues since he was very young. He had explosive tantrums as a toddler and was expelled from his first elementary school after striking another child. By 10, Tommy was suicidal. At the age of 12, he had first physically assaulted Linda, striking her when she tried to stop him from cutting himself. He started using drugs and alcohol at 13, and it was only a few months after this that Linda had called the police on her son during a drug-induced episode so bad she was afraid Tommy might try to kill himself or others. Since then, she has had to call the police to their home several times a year when she could no longer control Tommy.

Linda has done everything she can for her son. She is a part-time school psychologist on a limited income, and although Tommy qualifies for Medicaid, many of the services he has required over the years have not been covered by the government funded health care program. To complicate matters further, Linda and Tommy live in a relatively remote part of a state in the western United States. Access to mental health care in their part of the state is extremely limited, and for the sort of care Tommy has needed they have been required to travel to a city over three hours away. Tommy has been under the care of several psychologists and psychiatrists and has experienced brief psychiatric holds, but the company that manages Tommy's Medicaid funding has refused the expensive, months-long inpatient treatments his care providers have recommended. The one time that the insurance company approved treatment in an inpatient facility, they only approved spending half of what would be required for Tommy to stay at a facility in state. The closest juvenile facility that would accept Tommy at the funding provided was almost a thousand miles away. When Linda dropped him off at the out-of-state facility, she was appalled at the conditions. It was dirty and it seemed like the residents were not provided with sufficient supervision. When she received a phone call from Tommy three weeks later saying that he was in the infirmary after two other residents beat him up, Linda called state child protective services on the facility and brought Tommy home. Child protective services investigated and found that Tommy had experienced abuse at the hands of several other residents.

Linda has taken out private loans to secure Tommy's treatment in other facilities when she could. She has even brought his case to the attention of the local media in an attempt to shame the insurance company into funding the care he needed. Nothing has been enough, and Linda despairs of ever being able to get Tommy the treatment he needs.

Two nights ago, Linda called the police again on her son, but this time was different. High and angry, Tommy had lunged at Linda with a knife and struck her repeatedly across the face. The police came and brought Tommy to the Emergency Department where he was admitted for the night, but no juvenile psychiatric beds were available for Tommy. Linda was called to pick him up and she refused, explaining she was afraid her son would kill her and that she knew the hospital would be forced to care for him if no guardian would claim him.

Linda wonders what to do. She knows that by refusing to bring Tommy home, she faces the possibility of charges of child neglect. She also fears that giving up all parental rights and relinquishing custody of Tommy to the state is the only way to get Tommy the treatment he needs. She's not sure if she would be able to have contact with Tommy if she does so, though, or if she would ever be able to regain custody of her son.

Questions

1. What do you think Linda should do in this difficult situation?
2. What aspects of the U. S. medical system are contributing to the problems described in this case? What options are available to Linda? What should she do?
3. Although federal law requires parity in insurance coverage for "medically necessary" physical and mental health medical services, in practice, those without private insurance or with insufficient private

insurance often are unable to receive necessary mental health services. For those on government-provided health insurance, states define "medically necessary" coverage differently, which makes receiving mental health care in some states much harder than others. Should there be a federally mandated definition of "medically necessary" mental health care? If so, how would you go about defining what was medically necessary mental health care?

Resources

Bringewatt, Elizabeth H., and Elizabeth T. Gershoff. "Falling through the Cracks: Gaps and Barriers in the Mental Health System for America's Disadvantaged Children." *Children and Youth Services Review* 32, no. 10 (2010): 1291–99. https://doi.org/10.1016/j.childyouth.2010.04.021.

Cooper, Janice L., Yumiko Aratani, Jane Knitzer, Ayana Douglas-Hall, Rachel Masi, Patti L. Banghart, and Sarah Dababnah. "Unclaimed Children Revisited: The Status of Children's Mental Health Policy in the United States." Columbia Academic Commons. 2008. https://doi.org/10.7916/D8BR91XN.

Eckholm, Erik. "Nebraska Revises Child Safe Haven Law." *The New York Times*, November 21, 2008. https://www.nytimes.com/2008/11/22/us/22nebraska.html.

Herman, Christine. "To Get Mental Health Help For A Child, Desperate Parents Relinquish Custody." *NPR*, January 2, 2019. https://www.npr.org/sections/health-shots/2019/01/02/673765794/to-get-mental-health-help-for-a-child-desperate-parents-relinquish-custody.

Wan, William. "'Is This What a Good Mother Looks Like?'" *Washington Post*, March 17, 2022. https://www.washingtonpost.com/dc-md-va/2022/03/17/parental-rights-mental-illness-custody/.

6.5 Providing Care for a Frequent Visitor to the Emergency Room

Keywords: bias, homelessness, social determinants of health

Kenny W is a 59-year-old man with Type 2 diabetes. Kenny takes oral medication for diabetes and uses a glucometer to test blood sugar when he has access to lancets and strips. Kenny lives in a tent encampment, and he is food insecure. His poor diet and hygiene contribute to ongoing health issues, which he typically addresses by going to a nearby emergency room, where staff casually refer to him as a "frequent flier." When circumstances permit and he has access to transportation, Kenny also visits a community clinic on the other side of town for medical attention.

A few days after his last lancet stick, Kenny's index finger becomes swollen and painful, and he goes to the ER for treatment. Dr. M is new to the hospital, and she is seeing Kenny for the first time. Dr. M drains the abscess and provides antibiotics. She also provides Kenny with alcohol wipes to clean his fingers before and after sticks, to hopefully prevent future infections. She schedules a follow-up appointment at the community clinic in 10 days and calls in a social worker for consultation. The social worker chats with Kenny and offers him a bed at a local shelter as well as access to a food assistance program.

Kenny declines the bed and does not make use of the food assistance program because he is unable to attend the required nutritional consultation and he cannot provide an address for food delivery. He also misses his follow-up appointment, due to lack of transportation. When the alcohol wipes run out, he stops checking his blood sugar, and soon returns to the Emergency Department feeling very ill. This time, he is seen by a veteran hospitalist, Dr. G, who diagnoses him with hyperglycemia and a urinary tract infection. Dr. G, who has seen Kenny several times before, prescribes antibiotics as well as fluids to address dehydration. Nurse C discusses the importance of hygiene with Kenny and provides him with a fresh supply of alcohol wipes. Kenny is discharged and returns to his camp.

After Kenny leaves, Dr. G tells Nurse C, who is new to the hospital, that she can plan on seeing him again in the next few weeks. "These people are stuck in an endless cycle. We do our best to help them, but they refuse services, fail to follow up, and almost always revert to unhealthy practices, especially drug use." Nurse C asks Dr. G whether there is more they can do to help people like Kenny, who are obviously living under challenging circumstances. Dr. G's response is matter of fact: "Not my job. I give him good care when he's here, but it is not my job to fix his life outside the hospital or solve the problems that plague his city."

Nurse C is troubled by this response, as it seems to be at odds with her recently completed ethics curriculum, which emphasized professional responsibilities to reduce health disparities, and to provide care that is attentive to the dignity, worth, and unique attributes of individuals. She is also concerned that Dr. G's dismissiveness may harbor a racial component, since Kenny, like most homeless persons in the community, is a person of color.

She wonders whether to bring this up with other members of the medical staff or administration.

Questions

1. What additional steps, if any, should Dr. G and Nurse C take to address the social conditions that are contributing to Kenny's health problems?

2. Do individual health care workers have a responsibility to address the social conditions that create health challenges and disparities for patients like Kenny? If not, why? If so, what should they do to fulfill this responsibility?

3. Do hospitals have a responsibility to address the social conditions that create health challenges and disparities for patients like Kenny? If not, why? If so, what should they do to fulfill this responsibility?

Resources

American Nursing Association. "Code of Ethics for Nurses." https://www.ius.edu/nursing/handbooks/pre-nursing-handbook/standards-of-performance/code-of-ethics.html

Gottlieb, Laura M., Stacy Tessler Lindau, and Monica E. Peek. "Why Add 'Abolition' to the National Academies of Sciences, Engineering, and Medicine's Social Care Framework." *AMA Journal of Ethics* 24, no. 3 (2022): E170–80. doi: 10.1001/amajethics.2022.170.

Guarav, Dave, Mary K. Wolfe, and Giselle Corbie-Smith. "Role of Hospitals in Addressing Social Determinants of Health: A Groundwater Approach." *Preventive Medicine Reports* 21 (2021): 101315. https://www.sciencedirect.com/science/article/pii/S2211335521000061?via%3Dihub

Reference

Adapted from Gottlieb, Laura M., Stacy Tessler Lindau, and Monica E. Peek. "Why Add 'Abolition' to the National Academies of Sciences, Engineering, and Medicine's Social Care Framework." *AMA Journal of Ethics* 24, no. 3 (2022): E170–80. doi: 10.1001/amajethics.2022.170.

6.6 Withholding Surgery from a Patient with a History of Nonadherence

Keywords: bias, heart disease, nonadherence, race

Jose R is a 52-year-old man with a wife and three children. Although Jose has lived most of his life in the United States, his English is at best moderately proficient. His health is also not so good. He has a history of hypertension, exacerbated by years of smoking and bouts of substance abuse. Despite his health challenges, Jose has managed to support his family through a series of jobs in construction.

In recent weeks, Jose has experienced periods of dizziness and shortness of breath, as well as some swelling in his ankles. Tests show that he has mitral valve stenosis, caused by rheumatic heart disease and hypertension. Jose is scheduled for a meeting with Dr. M, a cardiac surgeon at the medical center where he is being treated. Before his meeting with Jose, Dr. M carefully studies his medical file, and discovers Jose has a history of nonadherence, specifically regarding prescribed medications. A previous cardiologist notes that Jose often went off his blood pressure medication for extended periods of time, and his primary care physician notes that Jose also failed to take prescribed medications, including statins and antibiotics. A conversation with the primary care physician also reveals that Jose frequently missed appointments and failed to make "heart healthy" lifestyle changes. His diet remains poor and, although he has greatly reduced smoking, he still smokes cigars and an occasional cigarette.

This history of nonadherence is troubling to Dr. M and complicates his thinking about Jose's treatment options. Patients with mitral valve stenosis may be treated with a balloon valvuloplasty, a minimally invasive procedure that attempts to widen the narrowing in the valve, or valve replacement surgery, which is much more invasive. Dr. M sometimes recommends valve replacement for patients like Jose, because the surgery can improve long-term outcomes in his age group, but he is reluctant to consider this option for Jose. Valve replacement requires rigorous post-surgical monitoring and medication management, and he is not confident Jose will come to follow-up appointments or take his medications. Dr. M concludes that Jose is not a good candidate for valve replacement surgery and does not offer it as an option.

Questions

1. Does Jose's history of nonadherence justify Dr. M's decision to not offer valve replacement surgery?
2. If you think Dr. M should offer the option of valve replacement surgery, what steps should he take to address his concerns about Jose's history of nonadherence?
3. Suppose Jose needed a heart transplant rather than surgery. Do you think his history of nonadherence should be considered in deciding whether he should be put on the transplant list?
4. Do you think Jose's case raises concerns about social justice? If so, what are your main concerns and how might they be addressed?

Resources

Sandal, Shaifali, Tinyan Chen, and Marcelo Canatrovich. "Evaluation of Transplant Candidates with a History of Nonadherence: An Opinion Piece." *Canadian Journal of Kidney Health and Disease* 8 (2021): 1–7. https://doi.org/10.1177/2054358121990137

Tran, Nhi, Amina Kouyate, and Monica U. Hahn. "Why Professionalism Demands Abolition of Carceral Approaches to Patients' Nonadherence Behaviors." *AMA Journal of Ethics* 24, no. 3. (2022): E181–87. doi:10.1001/amajethics.2022.181

6.7 Repeat Heart Surgery for an IV Drug User

Keywords: addiction, bias, resource allocation

Kim M is a 26-year-old mother of two, who has been struggling with IV drug use since her late teens. Less than one year ago, Kim had open heart surgery to replace her tricuspid valve, which was damaged as a result of endocarditis, a serious infection caused by her drug use. Kim is now back in the hospital, gravely ill with another bout of endocarditis. The infection has severely damaged her replacement valve, and the only way to save her life is to install another valve.

Dr. M is the cardiac surgeon who is assessing Kim. After reviewing her medical history, he discusses the case with Dr. S, the hospitalist who is on call. Dr. M expresses serious reservations about performing the surgery. Kim obviously continued to use drugs after her previous surgery, which damaged her replacement valve, and Dr. M has no reason to think she will stop using drugs after another surgery. It is likely that she will contract endocarditis again, damaging the new replacement valve, requiring an additional surgery. Dr. M is also concerned about effective use of valuable resources. Kim is uninsured and is not eligible for Medicaid, which means the hospital will have to absorb the substantial cost of her surgery. Of course, the hospital's ability to absorb such costs is limited, and Dr. M believes their funds would be better spent on other needy patients who are more likely to benefit, including other heart patients who might need valve replacement surgeries. Dr. M says he could perhaps justify surgery if Kim agreed to enter a drug rehab facility, but he is not convinced she would agree to this condition and, even if she did, he is not sure if there is a bed available in a local rehab facility. His inclination is to tell Kim that she is not a good candidate for surgery and recommend comfort care as the best course of action.

Dr. S listens carefully to Dr. M's reasoning but expresses disagreement with his inclination to withhold the surgery. Dr. S points out that Kim is medically fit to handle the surgery, and he does not believe the decision should be based on whether she is likely to pursue a healthy lifestyle after surgery. He asks, only half joking, whether Dr. W would withhold surgery from patients who are likely to continue eating fried foods and ice cream after surgery, or who may continue smoking against medical advice.

Dr. S's comments give Dr. M cause for pause, and they decide to solicit input from the hospital's ethics committee.

Questions

1. Would Dr. M be justified in withholding heart surgery from Kim?
2. Would Dr. M be justified in setting conditions before authorizing heart surgery, such as mandatory postoperative drug treatment? Would he be justified in refusing future surgeries if Kim contracts endocarditis due to continued drug use? Should there be a limit on the number of repeat valve replacements for a patient due to recurrent drug use?
3. Who should decide whether patients like Kim should be eligible for multiple valve replacements? The attending physician? The hospital? The state? What factors should be considered in such decisions?
4. What role, if any, should resources play in this decision? Would effective stewardship of resources justify denying surgery to Kim? Suppose Kim was a successful celebrity with money to pay for her own surgery. Would that affect your reasoning about whether she should receive multiple replacement surgeries?
5. Suppose resources are limited, and a rural facility has multiple patients in need of valve replacement surgery. Should the facility prioritize patients who are not IV drug users?

Resources

Ahmed, Talha and Ayesha Safdar, "Ethical Dilemma: Should Continuous Intravenous Drug Use Affect Appropriate Management in Prosthetic Valve Endocarditis?" *Cureus* 12, no. 6 (2020): e8458. Doi: 10.7759/cureus.8458.

Goodnough, Abby. "Injecting Drugs Can Ruin a Heart: How Many Second Chances Should an IV Drug User Get? *The New York Times*, April 29, 2018.

6.8 Ignoring the Symptoms of an Obese Patient

Keywords: bias, obesity

Reginald G is a certified nursing assistant in an ambulatory care clinic that has a primary care residency. He is on shift one day with Dr. W, a new resident who Reginald finds cocky and hard to work with.

Reginald completes an intake with a returning patient, Deborah H, who comes in complaining of a rash on her lower legs and joint pain. A notation in Deborah's chart indicates a history of weight issues and that Deborah is considered obese due to a body mass index of over 30. He tells Deborah he'll be back with the doctor in a moment and leaves to update Dr. W.

Dr. W and Reginald return to the room and Dr. W asks Deborah what brought her into the clinic. She explains about her rash and joint pain, and Dr. W cuts her off. "Joint pain is made much worse by being obese. Have you considered dieting?" It is clear Deborah is embarrassed by Dr. W's comment, and she mutters, "I have. Maybe that will help." Dr. W tells Deborah to increase her lean protein and vegetable intake and to start taking walks, and to come back in two months if she is not feeling better. He barely looks at the rash on her lower legs.

Reginald believes Deborah is being discriminated against because of her obesity. He feels like Dr. W has not adequately addressed Deborah's concerns and realizes Deborah is not going to advocate for herself.

Questions

1. Should Reginald intervene on behalf of Deborah? If so, how?
2. Do you think it is appropriate for Dr. W to mention Deborah's weight? If so, why? If not, do you think he should have approached the issue in a different way?
3. Polls indicate that some doctors refuse to treat obese patients, fearing complications and malpractice suits. Is this refusal ever ethical?
4. Do you think doctors and health care workers discriminate against people who are overweight? If so, how? What might be done to address such discrimination?

Resources

Kolata, Gina. "Why Do Obese Patients Get Worse Care? Many Doctors Don't See Past the Fat." *The New York Times*, September 26, 2016. https://www.nytimes.com/2016/09/26/health/obese-patients-health-care.html.

Phelan, S. M., D. J. Burgess, M. W. Yeazel, W. L. Hellerstedt, J. M. Griffin, and M. Ryn. "Impact of Weight Bias and Stigma on Quality of Care and Outcomes for Patients with Obesity." *Obesity Reviews* 16, no. 4 (2015): 319–26. https://doi.org/10.1111/obr.12266.

6.9 Talking with Patients about Weight Loss

Keywords: bias, obesity

Dr. M's second appointment of the day is a checkup with a long-term patient, Carol J. Carol is 46 and in relatively good health, though she has always fallen into the "overweight" or "obese" categories on body mass index (BMI) charts. Her BMI is currently 31.

The checkup goes well, and nothing seems amiss. When Dr. M asks Carol if she has any questions, Carol surprises her. "A friend of mine has been intermittent fasting and has lost a bunch of weight. She does not eat all day, and then eats whatever she wants from 4 pm until bedtime. I've been wondering whether I should do something similar, or at least try to go Keto."

Dr. M wonders how to respond. She knows the statistics on long-term weight loss: only 5 percent or less of those who lose weight will keep the weight off long term. She also knows that diets like Keto and intermittent fasting often have side effects and can be dangerous, and as such, Dr. M never recommends dieting to any patients. But she also knows that patients whose doctors are supportive of their weight loss goals tend to lose more weight, and that those who are overweight or obese tend to face considerably more stigma and discrimination than those who are thinner.

Questions

1. How should Dr. M respond to Carol? What questions should she ask and what recommendations should she make?

2. What are the ethical implications of recommending a course of action to patients (i.e., caloric restriction or dieting) that has low long-term efficacy?

3. What strategies and best practices should physicians use to facilitate fair and effective treatment of patients who are overweight?

Resources

Brown, Harriet. "The Weight of the Evidence." *Slate*, March 24, 2015. https://slate.com/technology/2015/03/diets-do-not-work-the-thin-evidence-that-losing-weight-makes-you-healthier.html.

Dimitrov Ulian, Mariana, Ana Jessica Pinto, Priscila de Morais Sato, Fabiana B. Bennati, Patricia Lopes de Campos-Ferraz, Desire Coelho, Odilon J. Roble, et al. "Effects of a New Intervention Based on the Health at Every Size Approach for the Management of Obesity: The 'Health and Wellness in Obesity' Study." Edited by Doan T. M. Ngo. *PLOS ONE* 13, no. 7 (2018): e0198401. https://doi.org/10.1371/journal.pone.0198401.

Prologo, J. David. "A Doctor's Open Apology to Those Fighting Overweight and Obesity." *The Conversation*, September 8, 2020. http://theconversation.com/a-doctors-open-apology-to-those-fighting-overweight-and-obesity-145017.

Tomiyama, A. Janet, Deborah Carr, Ellen M. Granberg, Brenda Major, Eric Robinson, Angelina R. Sutin, and Alexandra Brewis. "How and Why Weight Stigma Drives the Obesity 'Epidemic' and Harms Health." *BMC Medicine* 16, no. 1 (2018): 123. https://doi.org/10.1186/s12916-018-1116-5.

Tylka, Tracy L., Rachel A. Annunziato, Deb Burgard, Sigrún Daníelsdóttir, Ellen Shuman, Chad Davis, and Rachel M. Calogero. "The Weight-Inclusive versus Weight-Normative Approach to Health: Evaluating the Evidence for Prioritizing Well-Being over Weight Loss." *Journal of Obesity* (2014): 1–18. https://doi.org/10.1155/2014/983495.

6.10 Using Race in Clinical Algorithms

Keywords: bias, pain treatment, race

Luisa O is the Chief Diversity Office at Metropolitan Medical Center. In three years at Metropolitan, Luisa has increased minority hiring and helped implement educational workshops on cultural awareness and micro-aggressions. She is proud of her work, which she believes is having a tangible impact on the workplace.

One night over a glass of wine, her friend Anna tells her that she wishes Luisa could have an impact on discriminatory care at the Medical Center. Anna recounts the experience of her friend Jamaal, who had a difficult three-night stay at Metropolitan, during which he failed to receive adequate treatment for his post-operative pain. Jamaal suspects staff were inattentive to his requests for pain medications because he is African American. Luisa does not discount the possibility of implicit bias, but she tells Anna that pain management is complicated, and many doctors tend to undertreat pain because of concerns about addiction. Anna suggests that the problem is much deeper, citing studies that show African Americans are chronically undertreated for pain. Worse yet, physicians routinely employ clinical algorithms that adjust for race and, in so doing, decrease or delay referrals for specialized care for African Americans, particularly for kidney and heart disease. She offers to send Luisa links to these reports.

Luisa is deeply concerned after looking at these reports, and she approaches her supervisor, the Director of Human Resources, suggesting that she organize a workshop on racial biases in clinical algorithms. But the director does not respond favorably. He suggests that providing education on clinical algorithms is beyond her expertise, and that she should "stay in her lane," leaving clinical judgments to clinicians. If she receives evidence of discriminatory behavior by specific doctors, she should report that through the appropriate channels.

Luisa is disappointed in the director's response and ponders what to do next.

Questions

1. What additional steps, if any, should Luisa take to address her concerns about racial bias in clinical algorithms?
2. What problems arise when race is considered in diagnosis, prognosis, and treatment recommendations?
3. Should race ever be taken into account in clinical judgments? If so, when and how?
4. What initiatives and policies should be considered to help address racial inequities in our health care system?

Resources

Sederstrom, Nneka and Tamika Lasege. "Anti-Black Racism as a Chronic Condition." *Hastings Center Report* 52, no. 2 (2022): S24–29. https://doi.org/10.1002/hast.1364

Tong, Michelle and Samantha Artiga. "Use of Race in Clinical Diagnosis and Decision Making: Overview and Implications." Kaiser Family Foundation. December 9, 2021. https://www.kff.org/racial-equity-and-health-policy/issue-brief/use-of-race-in-clinical-diagnosis-and-decision-making-overview-and-implications/

Vyas, Darshali, Leo G. Eisenstein, and Daniel S. Jones. "Hidden in Plain Sight: Reconsidering the Use of Race Correction in Clinical Algorithms." *New England Journal of Medicine* 383, no. 9 (2020): 874–82. doi: 10.1056/NEJMms2004740.

6.11 Closing a Rural Primary Care Clinic

Keywords: resource allocation, rural health care

Dr. M is the Chief Medical Officer (CMO) at a small rural critical access hospital with twenty-five staffed beds. It is the only hospital in the county, as well as for the three surrounding counties. The hospital is also affiliated with two primary care facilities that Dr. M also oversees. As a CMO of a small hospital, Dr. M's responsibilities are many and varied. In addition to supervising the clinicians at the hospital and the primary care facilities, Dr. M is one of the chief points of contact for the board of directors of the hospital that oversees the budget and operations of the hospital.

The Chief Executive Officer of the hospital, Dr. X, approaches Dr. M one day looking sullen. Dr. X explains she just got off a call with the president of the board of directors who once again floated the idea of closing one of the two primary care facilities associated with the hospital. Between Medicare cuts and pandemic-related profit losses due to canceled elective procedures, the hospital is in worse financial straits than it has ever been. The primary care facility that the board members are considering closing has never made the hospital any money, but it is seen as part of the rural hospital's mission to provide care to the community of which they were a part. This facility is in the farthest reaches of the county, bordering another county that was served by the hospital, and the presence of this facility means many people do not need to travel a hundred miles for access to primary care. No one on the board or on hospital administration lives in the community the clinic is in, but they are aware that the facility and its clinicians are a deeply important part of the community, and the hospital has won recognition for providing access to primary care in such a remote location. Dr. X explains that the board members are distressed at the thought of closing the facility but need to protect the viability of both the hospital and the other primary care facility and see no other way to cut costs sufficiently to do so.

Questions

1. What steps should be taken before deciding whether to close the primary care facility? What facts are most relevant to this decision?

2. How should administrators and board members weigh the needs of a distant community and the hospital's mission against concerns about economic viability? What sort of information is necessary to make such judgments?

3. What role, if any, should the reputation of the hospital play in determining whether to close the primary care facility?

4. What initiatives and policies might be adopted to address the challenges associated with rural health care services?

Resources

American Hospital Association. *Final Recommendations: Future of Rural Health Care Task Force.* May 2021. https://www.aha.org/2021-05-17-final-recommendations-future-rural-health-care-task-force-may-2021.

Nelson, William A., ed. *Handbook for Rural Health Care Ethics: A Practical Guide for Professionals.* New Hampshire: Dartmouth College Press, 2009. https://geiselmed.dartmouth.edu/cfm/wp-content/uploads/sites/97/2022/04/full-book.pdf

Reference

Adapted from Nelson, William A., ed. *Handbook for Rural Health Care Ethics: A Practical Guide for Professionals,* 167–68. New Hampshire: Dartmouth College Press, 2009.

6.12 Medical Records in a Rural Setting

Keywords: confidentiality, rural health care

Jamie G is a 24-year-old woman who has lived in a small, rural town for her entire life, just as her parents and grandparents did before. The town only has 4,000 inhabitants and the community is very close. Jamie's family is well known by the inhabitants of town, and everywhere Jamie goes in town, she sees someone she knows. Jamie's doctor's office is no exception. Her cousin, Jessie, is the receptionist for her doctor, Dr. W. Jamie has been seeing Dr. W since she was a baby, and he has been a close friend of her family since before Jamie was born. Dr. W wears many hats given that he is the only one of two doctors practicing in town, so he also performs well-woman exams for those of his patients who do not have a separate gynecologist.

When Jamie goes in for her annual checkup and well-woman exam, Dr. W discovers an open lesion that he identifies as a genital herpes lesion. When he tells Jamie this, she becomes flustered and concerned. As his receptionist, Jessie handles all the documentation for Dr. W, including typing up medical records. Jamie wonders whether it is possible to keep the diagnosis of genital herpes out of her medical records since Jamie does not want Jessie to know.

Questions

1. Should Dr. W leave Jamie's genital herpes diagnosis out of her medical records?
2. Confidentiality in small communities can be extremely hard to maintain. Are there policies or procedures that Dr. W might enact that might help mitigate these concerns?

Resources

Medical Association of the State of Alabama (blog). "Delivery and Confidentiality Challenges in Rural Health Care Explained." June 13, 2019. https://alabamamedicine.org/the-delivery-and-confidentiality-challenges-in-rural-health-care-explained/.

Purtilo, Ruth and James Sorrell. "The Ethical Dilemmas of a Rural Physician." *Hastings Center Report* 16, no. 4 (1986): 24. https://doi.org/10.2307/3563112.

Townsend, Tom. "Patient Privacy and Mental Health Care in the Rural Setting." *AMA Journal of Ethics* 13, no. 5 (2011): 282–86. https://doi.org/10.1001/virtualmentor.2011.13.5.ccas3-1105.

Warner, Teddy D., Pamela Monaghan-Geernaert, John Battaglia, Christiane Brems, Mark E. Johnson, and Laura Weiss Roberts. "Ethical Considerations in Rural Health Care: A Pilot Study of Clinicians in Alaska and New Mexico." *Community Mental Health Journal* 41, no. 1 (2005): 21–33. doi: 10.1007/s10597-006-2597-1

Reference

Adapted from University of Montana. "The Healthcare Ethics Studies." https://www.umt.edu/bioethics/healthcare/resources/educational/casestudies/ruralfocus/confidentiality.aspx

6.13 Gender Affirming Hormones for an Adolescent

Keywords: autonomy, LGBTQ+ issues, minors, parental authority

Yorick S is a 13-year-old transgender boy who Dr. D, an endocrinologist, has been treating for five years. Although Yorick was born with genitalia that would indicate a feminine gender identity, Yorick and his parents report that he's said he has felt like a boy since about six. Yorick was diagnosed with gender dysphoria at seven years old. Gender dysphoria refers to distress or unease that is felt because of a discrepancy between a person's gender identity and the sex that person was assigned at birth. With the help of mental health professionals and doctors, the decision was made by Yorick and his parents for him to socially transition at eight years old, around the age when Dr. D started working with Yorick, and he started on puberty suppressing medication at 11 years old.

In the several years Dr. D has known Yorick, he has blossomed. He plays sports, joined the school band, has friends, and seems to be a well-liked and well-adjusted boy. His parents have kept him in therapy in order to make sure he's receiving the emotional support he needs and have been extremely supportive of their son's identity and transition.

Dr. D is surprised, then, when Yorick and his parents come to Dr. D's office visibly upset. Yorick's mom reports that she and her husband have been arguing with Yorick since his last appointment several months ago. Yorick wishes to begin gender-affirming hormone therapy so he can develop at approximately the same age as his peers, but his parents want him to wait until he turns 16, since they have read that this is the recommended age at which to start gender-affirming hormone therapy. They have come to Dr. D for advice.

Dr. D recognizes Yorick's parents only want to make sure to protect their son's health, and they're right that in the past, most adolescents started hormone therapy at around 16. Yet newly released guidelines put out by the World Professional Organization for Transgender Health have moved the recommended age to start gender-affirming hormone care to 14. Yorick's 14th birthday is only nine months away. Dr. D also knows that Yorick is a very mature young person whose gender identity has been stable for years. Yorick expresses concerns that he won't mature as fast as his friends and peers, physically or otherwise, if he stays on puberty blockers and waits too long to begin a hormone regimen. The physical side effects associated with gender-affirming hormone therapy remain the same at Yorick's current age or at 16.

Yorick is adamant about his desire to begin hormone therapy as soon as possible, and he asks Dr. D to help him do so even without his parent's consent.

Questions

1. If you were Dr. D, how would you advise Yorick and his parents? What sort of questions might you ask them?

2. Suppose Dr. D cannot facilitate agreement between Yorick and his parents. Should Dr. D consider starting Yorick on hormone therapy without his parents' consent?

Resources

Dubin, Samuel, Megan Lane, Shane Morrison, Asa Radix, Uri Belkind, Christian Vercler, and David Inwards-Breland. "Medically Assisted Gender Affirmation: When Children and Parents Disagree." *Journal of Medical Ethics* 46, no. 5 (2020): 295. https://doi.org/10.1136/medethics-2019-105567.

Ghorayshi, Azeen. "Doctors Debate Whether Trans Teens Need Therapy Before Hormones." *The New York Times*, January 13, 2022.

Kimberly, Laura L., Kelly McBride Folkers, Phoebe Friesen, Darren Sultan, Gwendolyn P. Quinn, Alison Bateman-House, Brendan Parent, et al. "Ethical Issues in Gender-Affirming Care for Youth." *Pediatrics* 142, no. 6 (2018): e20181537. https://doi.org/10.1542/peds.2018-1537.

6.14 Treating a Native American with Suicidal Tendencies

Keywords: addiction, social determinants of health, suicide

Dr. G is doing a residency rotation at an Indian Health Service (IHS) facility located on an impoverished rural reservation. Dr. G is a white man who was raised by two medical doctors who instilled in him a desire to serve medically underserved communities. After earning a Master's in Public Health, Dr. G decided to go to medical school and complete as much of his internal medicine residency in rural settings as possible.

One of Dr. G's first patients is Johnny, a 21-year-old Native American male who lives on the reservation where the IHS facility is located. Johnny has a history of narcotic use and has been brought to emergency departments twice for overdoses, including one last weekend. Johnny is in for a follow-up appointment after his release from the hospital. During their conversation, Dr. G learns that Johnny, like many young people on the reservation, is only marginally employed, never finished high school, and feels little hope about his future prospects. Johnny's girlfriend and mother of his son broke up with him two days before his last overdose and he's been couch surfing ever since. Dr. G begins to think that Johnny's accidental overdose may have actually been a suicide attempt. Dr. G is unsure of how to proceed. He's afraid if he even asks if Johnny is suicidal, he might alienate him and cause him to stop seeking medical care. Also, he is new to the clinic, but knows that in such a small community, word of how he treats Johnny will spread.

Questions

1. What should Dr. G do to help Johnny?
2. One of the options available to some health care professionals when they believe a patient is a danger to himself or others is an involuntary psychiatric hold, also known as a "5150." Assume it is established that Johnny is actively suicidal. Should Dr. G consider placing Johnny under an involuntary psychiatric hold to protect his welfare?
3. The problems experienced by Johnny are sadly common among persons living on reservations. What social and historical factors need to be taken into account to understand and treat patients like Johnny? Should Dr. G's treatment of Johnny differ from his approach to non-native patients with substance abuse problems and possible suicidal tendencies? If so, in what ways?
4. Many of the difficulties experienced by Johnny as described in this case are structural (i.e., resulting from social conditions beyond Johnny's control). What obligation, if any, do health care practitioners have to work toward solutions to structural issues that adversely impact the health and well-being of their patients?

Resources

Hasbah Roessel, M. "Working With Indigenous/Native American Patients." Psychiatry.Org. Accessed September 13, 2022. https://psychiatry.org:443/psychiatrists/diversity/education/best-practice-highlights/working-with-native-american-patients.

Oldani, Michael J. and Diedre Prosen. "Trauma-Informed Caring for Native American Patients and Communities Prioritizes Healing, Not Management." *AMA Journal of Ethics* 23, no. 6 (2021): E446–55. https://doi.org/10.1001/amajethics.2021.446.

Reference

Adapted from Oldani, Michael J. and Diedre Prosen. "Trauma-Informed Caring for Native American Patients and Communities Prioritizes Healing, Not Management." *AMA Journal of Ethics* 23, no. 6 (2021): E446–55. https://doi.org/10.1001/amajethics.2021.446

6.15 Suspected Abuse of an Adolescent Patient

Keywords: minor, parental authority, religion

Dr. V is a physician at a family practice clinic in a small mountain town of about 2,500 people in a rural area. Dr. V was born in the town and returned as soon as she finished her medical education. The town has always felt idyllic to Dr. V. Everyone knows everyone, and everyone looks out for each other. Because of winter ski tourism, the town is also faring better economically than many neighboring towns and her patients live generally stable lives.

Her first patient of the day is Angela P, a 15-year-old girl. Dr. V is surprised to see no previous medical records in Angela's chart when she goes to review Angela's records before seeing Angela.

When Dr. V enters the exam room, the first thing she notices is that Angela looks emaciated. Angela is 5'6", but she weighs only 95 pounds. With a body mass index (BMI) of 15.5, this puts her in the underweight category and given how low her BMI is, Dr. V wonders about malnutrition. Angela is also extremely withdrawn, folded into herself and reluctant to make eye contact. When Dr. V asks her what brings her to the office, Angela's father, Matt, answers for her. "She has a cough that won't go away. It's keeping her awake at night." Dr. V tries to find ways to get Angela to respond to her questions, but Matt keeps answering for his daughter. When asked about Angela's lack of medical records, Matt explains that his family moved to town recently and they haven't had any records transferred yet.

Dr. V begins to suspect that Matt and his family are part of a new religious settlement located northeast of town in the mountains. She has heard only rumors about the beliefs of the people in the community but understands that it is connected to the Christian Patriarchy movement, a movement that centers its theology around what the movement considers an Old Testament understanding of family and the differing roles of women and men. Under the Christian Patriarchy, fathers are granted absolute authority over their wives and children, and even any unmarried adult female children.

Dr. V explains to Matt and Angela that since this is Angela's first visit, she would like to conduct a full examination of Angela, and it might be better for Matt to leave the exam room. Matt refuses, saying, "My daughter has a cough. That's what she's here to be treated for and I am sure she is more comfortable with me in the room."

Dr. V wonders how to proceed. She fears if she pushes the issue, Matt might take his daughter and never return, but without the ability to ask Angela questions, Dr. V won't be able to ascertain why Angela is so underweight and whether abuse might be to blame. Unlike other cases in the past where Dr. V has suspected the neglect or abuse of a child, she sees no physical injuries on Angela, nor has medical records to establish patterns of abuse or neglect.

Questions

1. What would you do if you were Dr. V? How would you proceed with the examination?
2. In most states, physicians are considered mandatory reporters, which means they are required by law to report suspected child maltreatment or abuse. Since Dr. V has limited information regarding Angela and her situation, does she have a duty to inform local child protective services about this case?

Resources

Antommaria, Armand H. Matheny, Kathryn L. Weise, Mary E. Fallat, Aviva L. Katz, Mark R. Mercurio, Margaret R. Moon, Alexander L. Okun, and Sally A. Webb. "Conflicts Between Religious or Spiritual Beliefs and Pediatric Care: Informed Refusal, Exemptions, and Public Funding." *Pediatrics* 132, no. 5 (2013): 962–65. https://doi.org/10.1542/peds.2013-2716.

Christian, Cindy W., Committee on Child Abuse and Neglect. "The Evaluation of Suspected Child Physical Abuse." *Pediatrics* 135, no. 5 (2015): E1337–54. https://doi.org/10.1542/peds.2015-0356.

St. Claire, Karen. "What To Do When It Might Be Child Abuse." *AMA Journal of Ethics* 11, no. 2 (2009): 111–16. https://doi.org/10.1001/virtualmentor.2009.11.2.ccas2-0902.

6.16 Drug Testing Prisoners without Their Consent

Keywords: addiction, consent, prisoners, privacy

Dr. M is a physician at a state-run prison. He has worked in the prison system for a few months now and is slowly learning the ins and outs of carceral health care. He is bothered by the broad language in the Health Insurance Portability and Accountability Act (HIPPA) that allows for the disclosure of personal health information of prisoners without consent and worries about some of the injuries he treats and the violence the prisoners are subjected to, but he is glad to be able to offer medical treatment to a vulnerable population.

Dr. M reports to the Warden of the prison, Warden H. Although he has not worked with the Warden for long, Dr. M gets the sense that the Warden keeps a very close eye on the things happening in his prison. He is not all that surprised then, when after a number of fentanyl-related overdoses occur within the facility, Warden H comes to ask Dr. M to consider running drug tests on whoever happens to visit the prison clinic and count these tests toward the prison's random drug-testing requirements. Warden H explains that he needs to find out who is distributing drugs in the prison and one of the quickest ways to do it is to find someone who is using them and pressure them into informing on the person distributing. Only when the supply is cut off, claims Warden H, will the overdoses stop happening.

Dr. M is sympathetic to the Warden's desire of ending the overdoses, but he is worried about testing all patients without cause or consent. He wonders whether his role as a doctor is being co-opted for penal and law enforcement goals.

Questions

1. How should Dr. M respond to the Warden's request? Would complying with the request compromise his duties as a physician?
2. The Warden sees clear benefits of testing, which Dr. M appreciates. Are there potential risks or negative consequences that might result from the proposed testing?
3. In what circumstances, if any, should prisons conduct drug testing on prisoners without their consent? What rules should govern drug testing of prisoners?
4. If an inmate tests positive for a drug test, how should the prison respond?

Resources

Kipnis, Kenneth. "Social Justice and Correctional Health Services." In *Medicine and Social Justice,* edited by Rosamond Rhodes, Margaret Battin, and Anita Silvers, 373–84. New York: Oxford University Press, 2012. https://doi.org/10.1093/acprof:osobl/9780199744206.003.0032.

Pont, Jörg, Stefan Enggist, Heino Stöver, Brie Williams, Robert Greifinger, and Hans Wolff. "Prison Health Care Governance: Guaranteeing Clinical Independence." *American Journal of Public Health* 108, no. 4 (2018): 472–76. https://doi.org/10.2105/AJPH.2017.304248.

Zraik, Karen. "New York Prisons Punish 1,600 Based on Faulty Drug Tests, Report Finds." *The New York Times,* January 22, 2022.

6.17 Race and Medical School Admissions

Keywords: bias, race

For the last 20 years, University Medical School has utilized a "holistic review" rubric to select which students will be admitted. In addition to academic performance, this rubric takes into account the experiences and attributes of applicants, including their racial, ethnic, and socioeconomic background. The use of holistic review is grounded in U Med's mission to train physicians who will serve persons in medically underserved communities. These communities are defined by inequitable health outcomes, and they are populated primarily by persons of color. Since it started using holistic review, U Med has admitted and graduated many more students who identify as Black or Hispanic, and some of these have started practices in the state's underserved communities.

Professor T, a new member of the admissions committee who has recently moved from another state, is surprised to learn that race and ethnicity are part of U Med's selection process. At his previous school, admissions committees were prohibited from considering these attributes. Professor T is especially uneasy about the racial and ethnic components of the holistic review rubric, arguing that taking minority students over those with stronger MCAT scores and GPAs might lead to more students "washing out" of their program. He also suggests that this aspect of the rubric is unfair to applicants who do not fall into underrepresented groups, but who nevertheless worked hard to achieve their dream of becoming a physician. Professor T asks the committee to reconsider these elements of the rubric, in order to promote both academic success and fairness.

Questions

1. How would you address Professor T's concerns about academic success and fairness? Do you think these concerns warrant eliminating race and ethnicity from the rubric?

2. What are the strongest arguments in favor of holistic review? Do you think holistic review is likely to yield better physicians? If so, how?

3. How, if at all, should medical schools take race and ethnicity into account in medical school admissions policies?

Resources

Blake, Valerie. "Affirmative Action and Medical School Admissions." *AMA Journal of Ethics* 14, no. 12 (2012): 1003–07. doi: 10.1001/virtualmentor.2012.14.12.hlaw1-1212

Lee, Rosa. "How Should Medical School Admissions Drive Health Care Workforce Diversity? *AMA Journal of Ethics* 23, no. 12 (2021): E912–18. doi: 10.1001/amajethics.2021.912

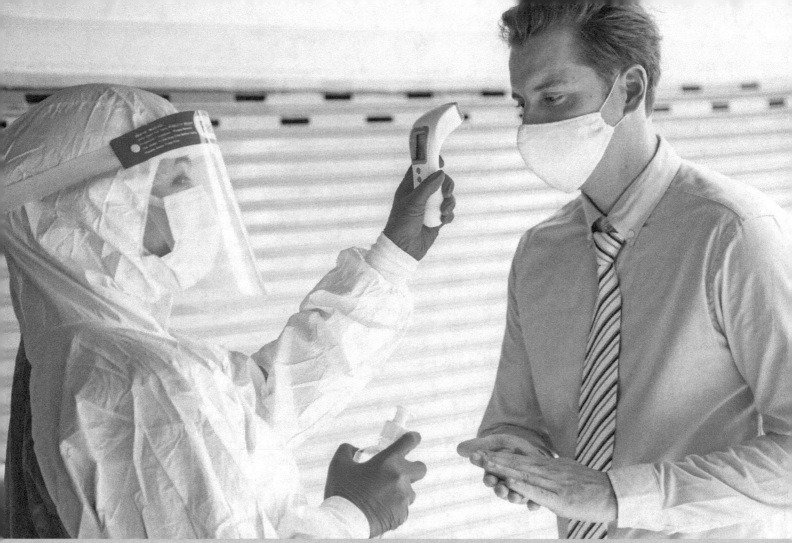

CHAPTER 7

Public Health Ethics

7.1 A Parent Refuses to Vaccinate

Keywords: parental authority, pediatrics, vaccines

A 5-year-old girl is brought into Dr. A's clinic by her mother for a wellness check and a pre-kindergarten visit. The child is a new patient. While conversing with the mother, Dr. A discovers that the family is transferring care to him after being told by their previous doctor that his practice will not care for children whose families do not vaccinate. The child is doing well and her exam is normal. Dr. A suggests a round of vaccinations for the child, explaining the benefits and risks, and asks if the mother has any questions. She has no questions, but she refuses to consent to vaccinations for her child. She asks Dr. A to fill out a form that certifies he has counseled the family about vaccinations. This form is necessary for the girl to enroll in public school.

Dr. A is conflicted over whether to sign the form, because he is concerned about the child's susceptibility to illness, and he is also concerned about a downward trend in vaccination rates in local schools, particularly for measles. Also, his practice includes "quality incentive" payments from a major insurance company, which depend in part on the vaccination rates of his patients. He decides to sign the form but wonders whether he is complicit in jeopardizing the health of his patient and other children.

Questions

1. What additional steps, if any, should the doctor take to persuade the mother to vaccinate her child?
2. Should the doctor sign the verification of counselling form? If he signs the form, does this make him complicit in harm to his patients and others if a measles breakout occurs?
3. Would the doctor be justified if, like the previous doctor, he decides to dismiss the patient? What role, if any, should the quality incentive play in the doctor's decision?
4. Several states in the United States only allow medical exemptions to mandatory vaccination requirements for children in public schools, while others allow philosophical and/or religious exemptions. Which exemptions do you think should be allowed?

Resources

Centers for Disease Control and Prevention. "Measles Data and Statistics." https://www.cdc.gov/measles/downloads/measlesdataandstatsslideset.pdf

Hoffman, Jan. "Measles Deaths Soared Worldwide Last Year, as Vaccine Rates Stalled." *The New York Times*, November 28, 2020. Updated October 28, 2021.

Politi, Mary C., Katherine M. Jones, and Sydney E. Philpott. "The Role of Patient Engagement in Addressing Parents' Perceptions about Vaccinations." *Journal of the American Medical Association* 318, no. 3 (2017): 237–38. doi:10.1001/jama.2017.7168.

7.2 Mandatory Vaccinations for Health Care Workers

Keywords: autonomy, COVID-19, vaccines

Dr. F is an intensivist and the Chief Medical Officer for a 200-bed midsized hospital in a small city. His hospital is the largest in a 150-mile radius, so although the hospital is not large, it receives most of the critically ill patients from the surrounding counties and bordering states. Dr. F's hospital has played a particularly important role in the region during the COVID-19 pandemic. During the worst point of the pandemic for the region so far, the hospital expanded capacity by 25 percent to deal with the number of people in the region who required hospitalization. They operated at surge capacity for a few weeks, and after the surge staff were exhausted and many had fallen ill with the disease. A particularly beloved nurse at the hospital who had been approaching retirement caught COVID-19 and died in the ICU in the hospital. Morale has been low among Dr. F's staff.

Dr. F has been feeling hopeful, however, as he watches the development of several vaccines that look promising. If the news is correct, one or more of the vaccines will receive emergency-use authorization from the Federal Drug Administration any day and should be available for frontline health care workers in a few short weeks. The initial trials on the vaccines are very promising. They appear to do much to prevent spread of the disease, but more importantly, the vaccines usually prevent hospitalization and death when a person contracts the disease. He hopes this news will boost the morale of his staff, especially the news that it's likely his staff will receive these lifesaving vaccines so soon.

When Dr. F announces that vaccine distribution will begin soon, he is surprised to learn that not everyone is excited about this prospect. Some of the nursing supervisors approach him and tell him some of their nurses would prefer not to receive the vaccine and are afraid about what it might mean for their jobs. Dr. F knows that vaccination might become mandatory for staff in the next few months but had not considered that the policy would be a practical necessity. He thought the devastation his staff had seen would make them as excited about receiving the vaccine as he is. He wonders how to address reluctance among some of his staff.

Questions

1. How should Dr. F proceed? What steps, if any, should he take to encourage vaccination? Should vaccination be mandatory in this case?

2. Under what circumstances, if any, should health care professionals be required to get vaccines?

3. Federal law allows employees to request exemption from vaccination based on "sincerely held religious belief," but it does not require health care institutions to accommodate this request if it creates "undue hardship." How would you assess whether a health care worker's request for a religious exemption from a vaccine is "sincere" and whether "undue hardship" might justify refusing such a request?

4. Some states do not allow a religious exemption for school children who want to attend public schools without being vaccinated. Do you think hospitals should be allowed to remove the religious exemption as well?

Resources

American Hospital Association. "CMS Issues Rule Requiring Mandatory Covid-19 Vaccinations for Health Care Workers." Special Bulletin. November 4, 2021. https://www.aha.org/special-bulletin/2021-11-04-cms-issues-interim-final-rule-requiring-mandatory-Covid-19-vaccinations.

Barnard, Anne, Grace Ashford, and Neil Vigdor. "These Health Care Workers Would Rather Get Fired Than Get Vaccinated." *The New York Times*, September 26, 2021.

Olick, Robert S., Jana Shaw, and Y. Tony Yang. "Ethical Issues in Mandating COVID-19 Vaccination for Health Care Personnel." *Mayo Clinic Proceedings* 96, no. 12 (2021): 2958–62. https://doi.org/10.1016/j.mayocp.2021.10.020.

7.3 COVID-19 Triage and Fairness

Keywords: bias, COVID-19, race, resource allocation, social determinants of health

Melanie K has been a medical ethicist on her state's Disaster Medical Advisory Committee for four years, the last six months of which have been during the COVID-19 respiratory pandemic. She and the committee members have been tasked with creating statewide guidance for how to triage scarce resources in emergency and acute settings. The state wants to ensure that decision-making is consistent across hospitals and geographic regions, and that the guidance finds ways to eliminate as much provider bias as possible from decisions regarding allocation of scarce resources. Most of the committee members only have clinical training, and no one other than Melanie has serious training in ethics.

As conversations around developing an algorithm for making triage decisions continue, most members of the committee insist that only "medically relevant" data be included in the information considered when determining who might receive a resource. Although much is still unknown about the novel virus, what is clear is that there are several comorbidities that usually lead to much worse short-term and long-term outcomes and are predictive of death at much higher rates in those that have them than the general population when one contracts the virus. These comorbidities include things like chronic kidney disease and diabetes, which Melanie knows that BIPOC populations, specifically black people and African Americans, suffer from at disproportionate rates because of social determinants of health. When her fellow committee members suggest that the primary criteria for receiving a scarce resource be tied to the absence of these comorbidities in a patient, she balks and explains why heavy reliance on these comorbidities might further exacerbate health inequities.

"But the point of triage is to save the most lives, Melanie," responds the intensivist who runs the committee. "That is our charge here: to save as many people as possible."

Questions

1. In traditional triage ethics, emphasis is often placed on saving the most lives or number of life years. Do you think this utilitarian approach is justified?

2. If you do not support the traditional utilitarian model, what alternative would you propose?

3. Should triage decisions be based only on "medically relevant data"? Does this approach reduce provider bias and promote fairness?

Resources

American Public Health Association. "Public Health Code of Ethics." https://www.apha.org/-/media/files/pdf/membergroups/ethics/code_of_ethics.ashx

Schmidt, Harald, Dorothy E. Roberts, and Nwamaka D. Eneanya. "Rationing, Racism and Justice: Advancing the Debate around 'Colourblind' COVID-19 Ventilator Allocation." *Journal of Medical Ethics* 48, no. 2 (2022): 126–30. doi:10.1136/medethics-2020-106856.

Tolchin, Benjamin, Sarah C. Hull, and Katherine Kraschel. "Triage and Justice in an Unjust Pandemic: Ethical Allocation of Scarce Medical Resources in the Setting of Racial and Socioeconomic Disparities." *Journal of Medical Ethics* 47, no. 3 (2021): 200–202. doi:10.1136/medethics-2020-106457.

White, Douglas B., and Bernard Lo. "Mitigating Inequities and Saving Lives with ICU Triage during the COVID-19 Pandemic." *American Journal of Respiratory Critical Care Medicine* 203, no. 3 (2021): 287–95. doi: 10.1164/rccm.202010-3809CP

7.4 Rationing CPR for COVID-19 Patients

Keywords: cardiopulmonary resuscitation, code status, COVID-19, futility

Maya M is a critical care nurse at a large hospital in New York City. It's January of 2021, and the hospital is experiencing a surge of COVID-19 patients. Although the pandemic has been raging in the United States for more than 10 months, few treatments are available, and workers are still facing a critical shortage of personal protective equipment (PPE). Best estimates suggest that more than 2,000 health care workers have died in the United States since the start of the pandemic and many more have fallen ill. The hospital is facing a critical shortage of staff and is having a hard time handling the influx of patients.

The nurses at Maya's hospital are committed to patient care, but they are also exhausted and concerned that the hospital is not sufficiently attentive to their own welfare. Especially frustrating is the lack of PPE, which is causing staff to reuse masks that were intended for single use. They are further demoralized by the recent deaths of two colleagues from COVID-19. In order to protect themselves, several of Maya's colleagues quietly decide to be more judicious in the use of cardiopulmonary resuscitation (CPR) for COVID-19 patients. Hospital protocols call for all patients who go into cardiac arrest to receive CPR, except those who have a Do-Not-Resuscitate order (DNR). Most patients do not have a DNR, so nurses are regularly called upon to provide CPR for seriously ill COVID-19 patients. Performing CPR brings significant risk of contagion to providers, and nurses know that outcomes are very poor, especially for elderly patients with severe comorbidities. So, several nurses decide to do "slow codes" on these severely ill patients; that is, they deliberately slow their response to code alerts, by taking their time when donning gowns and shields that are used during the procedure. This delay often means patients die before CPR is administered, saving nurses from needless exposure.

Maya is sympathetic to the plight of her colleagues, but she is also troubled by their actions. She is worried about unauthorized deviation from hospital protocol, and she wonders whether nurses should be taking it upon themselves to make these life and death decisions.

Questions

1. Are the nurses justified in rationing CPR, by focusing on patients who have better outcomes? If so, what are the key factors that justify this rationing? If not, what are your main reasons for opposing this action?
2. How should health care workers balance duties to others with risks to themselves? Do health care workers have a duty to provide patient care even when they lack appropriate PPE?
3. Under what circumstances and subject to what guidelines is rationing of care justified during a pandemic?
4. Statistics show that COVID-19 illness and deaths disproportionately affected nursing staff and assistants in comparison to physicians, and disproportionately impacted the persons of color in comparison to white persons. How, if at all, does that information affect your reasoning about rationing and resource allocation during the pandemic?

Resources

Catholic Health Association of the United States. "Code Status and COVID-19 Patients." www.chausa.org/docs/default-source/ethics/cha_scc_guidelines–final.pdf?sfvrsn=b9e0f5f2_0

Ciaffa, Jay. "The Ethics of Unilateral Do-Not-Resuscitate Orders for COVID-19 Patients." *Journal of Law, Medicine and Ethics* 49 (2021): 633–40.

Penn Medicine, Palliative and Advanced Care Research Center. "Crisis Standards of Care and Resource Allocation: Resources for Hospitals and Clinicians." April 2021. https://pair.upenn.edu/covid19/crisis-standardsofcare

7.5 A COVID-19 Positive Health Care Worker

Keywords: COVID-19, nursing

Nurse K works in an acute care unit at a suburban hospital in Florida, and she tested positive for a break-through COVID-19 infection four days ago. She is still symptomatic and is experiencing fever, a cough, and considerable fatigue. This is not the first time she has been sick with COVID-19. The first time was early in the pandemic when much less was known about how COVID-19 spread. At that time, she was required to stay at home from work for seven days and be without fever for five of those days.

Nurse K receives a phone call from her nursing administrator telling her to come into work the next day. Her administrator tells her that recently revised Centers for Disease Control guidelines have shifted to a five-day isolation period, and the guidelines indicate that hospital workers who test positive and whose symptoms are relatively mild and resolving could come back to work in five days. There are severe hospital staffing shortages across the city. The administrator explains that the hospital is close to being at nurse-to-patient ratios that would violate even the higher ratios allowed by the state during the COVID-19 pandemic, so the hospital really needs every available nurse at work. Staffing ratios, especially for nurses, have been extremely high and Nurse K knows that it is affecting patient care. She feels a duty to care for her patients, but also knows that it is likely she is still contagious and, given how sick she still feels, she will not be at her best as a nurse. She wonders whether returning to work is in the best interest of patients.

Questions

1. Should Nurse K cede to her administrator's request and go to work?
2. Suppose Nurse K's administrator told her that she would be assigned to the COVID-19 ward. Does this impact your reasoning about whether she should go to work?
3. How should health care workers balance concerns about their own well-being against the duty to care for patients? Does the welfare of patients always take precedence? If not, when, and how is it limited by concerns about the welfare of workers?

Resources

McDougall, Rosalind J., Lynn Gillam, Danielle Ko, Isabella Holmes, and Clare Delany. "Balancing Health Worker Well-Being and Duty to Care: An Ethical Approach to Staff Safety in COVID-19 and Beyond." *Journal of Medical Ethics* 47, no. 5 (2021): 318–23. https://doi.org/10.1136/medethics-2020-106557.

Nelson, Katie E. and Cynda Hylton Rushton. "Working While Ill During COVID-19: Ethics, Guilt, and Moral Community." *AACN Advanced Critical Care* 32, no. 3 (2021): 356–61. https://doi.org/10.4037/aacnacc2021342

7.6 Mandatory A1C Reporting

Keywords: privacy, surveillance

Dr. G, a physician who works for the public health department of a midsized city in the Midwestern United States, was flummoxed. He has just made a proposal to his city's board of health to develop a program modeled on New York City's A1C Registry (NYCAR) program, which requires laboratories with electronic reporting capabilities to submit data to the health department regarding A1C test results, a common blood test to diagnose Type 1 and Type 2 diabetes. The information reported to this program includes the A1C test results, the name and contact information of the person tested, their date of birth, and any available information on their primary physician. NYCAR serves two functions: tracking the prevalence of diabetes in the community through the examination of aggregate data, and informing clinicians of patients whose A1C results are poor. NYCAR has been especially useful in tracking Type 2 diabetes in children and helping public health officials design targeted interventions.

Dr. G expected the potential benefits of such a registry to be obvious to the board, but he receives immediate pushback.

"This feels like more government overreach. I don't want public health to have access to my medical information," says Steve, a local businessman recently appointed to the board of health.

"I'm not as concerned about government overreach, but I do have some concerns about privacy," responds Dr. M, a chiropractor who is a long-time member of the board. "It seems to me that it's harder to justify the invasion of privacy this registry would require given that diabetes isn't communicable."

Dr. J, the chair of the board of health and the dean of a medical college located in the city chimes in: "It's been considered part of public health's mission for some time now to focus on all potential sources of disease that cause mortality and morbidity, Dr. M, not just communicable diseases. This seems like a program that could help us understand where in our city we need to concentrate our diabetes prevention efforts."

Questions

1. What are the most significant concerns about privacy associated with Dr. G's proposal? What might be done to ameliorate these concerns?

2. Should the board of health institute a surveillance program like the one described? What steps should they take to determine whether it is an appropriate program for their city?

3. Do you support public health tracking of noncommunicable diseases? If not, why? If so, on what grounds?

Resources

Barnes, Clarissa, Frederick Brancati, and Tiffany Gary. "Mandatory Reporting of Noncommunicable Diseases: The Example of The New York City A1C Registry (NYCAR)." *AMA Journal of Ethics* 9, no. 12 (2007): 827–31. https://doi.org/10.1001/virtualmentor.2007.9.12.pfor2-0712.

Barrett, Drue, Leonard Ortmann, Angus Dawson, Carla Saenz, Andreas Reis, and Gail Bolan. eds. *Public Health Ethics: Cases Spanning the Globe,* 51–54. New York, NY: Springer Berlin Heidelberg, 2015.

Chamany, Shadi, Lynn D. Silver, Mary T. Bassett, Cynthia R. Driver, Diana K. Berger, Charlotte E. Neuhaus, Namrata Kumar, and Thomas R. Frieden. "Tracking Diabetes: New York City's A1C Registry." *Milbank Quarterly* 87, no. 3 (2009): 547–70. https://doi.org/10.1111/j.1468-0009.2009.00568.x.

7.7 HIV Surveillance in Commercial Sex Workers

Keywords: surveillance

Nurse M works for the Public Health Department in the large city in which she resides. She works in the Disease Control Department and engages with populations that are at high risk of sexually transmitted infections (STIs), providing STI testing, treatment, and prevention education in a mobile clinic. Nurse M has developed trusting relationships with her patients over the years, many of whom are living on the streets and doing sex work in order to survive.

Nurse M's boss sends out a memorandum one day about a new surveillance program involving commercial sex workers. The Public Health Department has conducted surveillance on the prevalence of HIV in the city for years but has never focused on data collection on sex workers specifically. The memorandum explains that incidence of STIs among sex workers is high and cites studies that indicate targeted intervention programs for sex workers on STI prevention and treatment have been effective in reducing the incidence of STIs. The Public Health Department will begin tracking data on HIV rates among commercial sex workers specifically in order to measure the impact of the new intervention program over time.

Nurse M has several concerns about this program. Although she understands the importance of data collection for measuring the effectiveness of interventions, she recognizes that including the designation of "commercial sex worker" on any patient file comes with significant risks to the patient. Prostitution is illegal in the state where Nurse M lives. She knows that first time offenders are charged with a misdemeanor and can be punished with three months in prison. Repeat offenders can be charged with a felony and sentenced to years in prison. For those who have HIV and engage in sex work, even the first offense can be charged as a felony. Since state law requires that health care providers provide the names of those who test positive for HIV to the state Department of Health, Nurse M worries about the implications of this sort of surveillance for both the patients she sees and the trust she's developed with them over the years.

Questions

1. What are the potential benefits to a surveillance program like the one described? What are the most significant potential risks? What might be done to limit these risks?
2. Given the criminality of prostitution, should the Public Health Department conduct surveillance of the incidence of HIV among sex workers? What impact, if any, should criminality have on data collection in public health?
3. What other agencies and groups should be involved in developing the new intervention program? What public and private stakeholders should be consulted?

Resources

Fairchild, Amy L., Ali Akbar Haghdoost, Ronald Bayer, Michael J. Selgelid, Angus Dawson, Abha Saxena, and Andreas Reis. "Ethics of Public Health Surveillance: New Guidelines." *The Lancet Public Health* 2, no. 8 (2017): E348–49. https://doi.org/10.1016/S2468-2667(17)30136-6.

Lou, Nina. "Decriminalizing Survival: Policy Platform and Polling on the Decriminalization of Sex Work." Data for Progress, 2020. https://www.filesforprogress.org/memos/decriminalizing-sex-work.pdf.

Shaver, Frances M. "Sex Work Research: Methodological and Ethical Challenges." *Journal of Interpersonal Violence* 20, no. 3 (2005): 296–319. https://doi.org/10.1177/0886260504274340.

7.8 Tracking Down a TB Patient

Keywords: addiction, confidentiality, nonadherence, privacy, quarantine

Dr. J is the health officer for a local health district in a county in California. One of the programs he oversees in this role is an opioid treatment program that uses a medication-assisted withdrawal approach to treatment. In addition to this, the program offers many wraparound services for those it serves, including medication management for diseases disproportionately experienced by intravenous drug users and those who experience homelessness, such as HIV and tuberculosis (TB).

One of the managers of the program, Drea H, comes to Dr. J about a client, Nick W, who has stopped coming into the clinic. Nick has been in and out of treatment for his addiction a lot over the years, so his stopping treatment is nothing new. What is new is his diagnosis of TB. In addition to receiving medication to help with his addiction, Nick has been receiving treatment for TB and is six weeks into a six-month treatment regimen. Although Nick's symptoms have greatly abated in his weeks on the antibiotic regimen, he still has a cough and complains of chest pains. Nick is very likely still contagious, and his discontinuation of the antibiotics will likely lead him to get much sicker. Drea worries that if they don't track down Nick to get him his antibiotics, he'll spread TB.

Drea reminds Dr. J that Nick is a member of a small community of Marshallese in their county. This is a tight-knit community, formed by persons who had to relocate in the 1960s after U.S. nuclear bomb testing rendered some of the Marshallese islands uninhabitable. This has left many of the Marshallese with a reasonable distrust of the government and governmental institutions. The health district has done its best to foster good relations with the Marshallese community and made a special effort to hire Marshallese workers.

It would likely be easy to find Nick if they could reach out to that community. Unfortunately, the only Marshallese caseworker in the county health office recently found a job elsewhere. Drea wonders whether it would be possible to reach out to the former caseworker who would be well positioned to make inquiries about Nick. Dr. J responds that a month before, it would have been no problem, because medical discussions with employees are permitted under HIPAA. Since the caseworker is no longer employed by the health district, Dr. J wonders whether he should reach out to him to help locate Nick.

Questions

1. What steps, if any, should Dr. J take to try to locate Nick?
2. Are there special considerations regarding confidentiality in this case given the small community of which Nick is a member? What are these special considerations?
3. Do public health professionals and organizations have a special responsibility toward communities that have suffered at the hands of the government? Why or why not? If so, what sort of special responsibilities exist?
4. Suppose Nick remains contagious and is not isolating himself from other people. What steps might be taken to protect others from contagion? Under what circumstances, if any, would you support forced isolation of persons who have infectious diseases such as TB?

Resources

Fidler, David P., Lawrence O. Gostin, and Howard Markel. "Through the Quarantine Looking Glass: Drug-Resistant Tuberculosis and Public Health Governance, Law, and Ethics." *Journal of Law, Medicine and Ethics* 35, no. 4 (2007): 616–28. https://doi.org/10.1111/j.1748-720X.2007.00185.x.

Night, Susan. "Public Health Emergencies and HIPAA: When Is the Disclosure of Individual Health Information Lawful?" *University of Houston Law Center* (2007). https://law.uh.edu/healthlaw/perspectives/2007/(SN)SpeakerHIPAA.pdf.

Parmet, Wendy E. "Legal Power and Legal Rights: Isolation and Quarantine in the Case of Drug-Resistant Tuberculosis." *New England Journal of Medicine* 357, no. 5 (2007): 433–35. https://www.nejm.org/doi/full/10.1056/nejmp078133

7.9 House Arrest to Prevent Spread of an Infectious Disease

Keywords: quarantine

Dr. M is a county health officer in a state in the southeastern United States. State law gives him the power to enforce quarantine for people who are carrying an infectious disease who refuse to self-quarantine, though, in his 15 years of being a county health officer, he has never needed to use this power. Unfortunately, a global respiratory pandemic caused by a novel virus has made its way to his county and state, which has now declared a state of emergency. Much is still unknown about the short- and long-term effects of respiratory disease. Best available data indicate that the mortality rate for adults is about 5 percent, though deaths tend to be concentrated among those over 50 and those in poor health. The county Dr. M serves in is an aging one; about 20 percent of his county's population is 65 or older.

Dr. M receives a phone call one night after work from Mr. N, an epidemiologist at the health department who is in charge of tracking positivity rates and positive cases in the county. Mr. N also oversees a program started to encourage self-quarantining after testing positive for the respiratory disease. The program asks those who test positive to sign self-quarantine documents that promise that they will not leave their residence for two weeks after they received their positive test result or five days after they are symptomatic, whichever is the longer term. Mr. N reports that a married couple in their mid-thirties is refusing to sign the self-quarantine documents because they are asymptomatic and do not wish to quarantine. Mr. N asks Dr. M what he should do.

Questions

1. How should Dr. M advise Mr. N? If the couple continues to refuse to quarantine, should Dr. M use his policing powers and place them under forced quarantine?

2. How does the fact that relatively little is known about the virus play into your reasoning about how Dr. M should respond to this couple's refusal to quarantine? Would your reasoning change if scientific studies confirmed the 5 percent mortality rate? Would your reasoning change if evidence showed a higher mortality rate?

3. The powers of public health officials to use state power coercively (e.g., through forced isolation and quarantine, inspection, and surveillance) are controversial, but often understood as necessary in order to protect public health in some instances. What ethical principles might justify the coercive use of state powers during a public health emergency? What principles might conflict with that use? When, if ever, would you support the use of forced quarantine?

Resources

American Bar Association, "Two Centuries of Law Guide Legal Approach to Modern Pandemic." 2020. https://www.americanbar.org/news/abanews/publications/youraba/2020/youraba-april-2020/law-guides-legal-approach-to-pandemic/.

Gostin, Lawrence O., and Lindsay F. Wiley. "Governmental Public Health Powers During the COVID-19 Pandemic: Stay-at-Home Orders, Business Closures, and Travel Restrictions." *Journal of the American Medical Association* 323, no. 21 (2020): 2137–38. https://doi.org/10.1001/jama.2020.5460.

Roberts, Abigail. "Kentucky Couple under House Arrest after Refusing to Sign Self-Quarantine Agreement." *ABC News*, July 20, 2020. https://abcnews.go.com/US/kentucky-couple-house-arrest-refusing-sign-quarantine-agreement/story?id=71886479.

Upshur, Ross. "The Ethics of Quarantine." *AMA Journal of Ethics* 5, no. 11 (2003): 393–95. https://doi.org/10.1001/virtualmentor.2003.5.11.msoc1-0311.

7.10 Resource Allocation and Racial Disparities

Keywords: race, resource allocation, social determinants of health

Dr. F is the medical director for the Public Health Department in a racially segregated urban city in the southeast with a high concentration of black Americans. One of the priorities for the department has been to decrease racial disparities in health outcomes that have long been part of the city's history. This priority has been woven throughout department programs, but one program that has been especially popular with the public has been focused on maternal-child health and the reduction of racial disparities in infant mortality. This program has been running for over a decade and a half, and in that time considerable improvement in black infant mortality has been seen, both nationally and locally.

General underfunding of public health has always been a problem during Dr. F's tenure as director, but recent budget cuts at the state level due to an economic downturn mean that some programs at the health department must be cut. Although the program focused on the reduction of racial disparities in infant mortality is a relatively inexpensive program and popular with the community, the effectiveness of the program has stalled over the last few years and the impact of the program on disparate rates of infant mortality seems to have waned. Other programs focused on other racially associated health disparities have met targets more consistently. Dr. F considers allocating the funds from the infant mortality program to other programs.

When Dr. F mentions this to Stacey, the director of community outreach, she suggests holding public forums to get feedback from the community on budget allocations. She reminds Dr. F how popular the program has been. Dr. F worries about the cost and time associated with community forums, however. Cuts need to be made relatively soon, and spending money on forums will make some of the budgeting issues worse.

Questions

1. Should Dr. F hold community forums to receive feedback on whether to reallocate the budget of the infant mortality program? What role should the community play in setting priorities for public health departments?

2. Does the waning effectiveness of the infant mortality program indicate that it no longer has value from a public health standpoint?

3. Do health departments have an obligation to reduce racial disparities? If so, does this obligation supersede the obligation to improve general public health metrics? How should these two obligations be balanced if and when they conflict?

4. What should be considered when allocating the resources to public health departments (e.g., community opinion, evidence-based practices, specific ethical principles)?

Resources

MacDorman, Marian F. and T.J. Mathews. "The Challenge of Infant Mortality: Have We Reached a Plateau?" *Public Health Reports* 124, no. 5 (2009): 670–81. https://doi.org/10.1177/003335490912400509.

Singh, Gopal K., and M. Yu Stella. "Infant Mortality in the United States, 1915-2017: Large Social Inequalities Have Persisted for Over a Century." *International Journal of Maternal and Child Health and AIDS* 8, no. 1 (2019): 19–31. https://doi.org/10.21106/ijma.271.

Reference

Adapted from Barrett, Drue H., Leonard W. Ortmann, Angus Dawson, Carla Saenz, Andreas Reis, and Gail Bolan, eds. *Public Health Ethics: Cases Spanning the Globe*. Vol. 3 (2016). Case 3.8.2, 85–86. https://www.ncbi.nlm.nih.gov/books/NBK435786/

7.11 Debating a Drop-In Center for Drug Users

Keywords: addiction

Dr. W is a primary care physician in a midwestern city with a population of 180,000. He has worked in his community for nearly 30 years, and he has seen a significant increase in opioid addiction over this time, accompanied by an alarming increase in overdose deaths. The city council has called a community meeting to discuss the problem. Dr. W is invited to speak at this meeting, since he has treated numerous patients who struggle with addiction and witnessed firsthand the devastating effects of the opioid crisis.

Dr. W begins his comments by saying that he thinks it's time to start thinking "outside the box" to address the opioid crisis in their community. He goes on to describe harm reduction programs that are showing positive results in other parts of the country. These programs feature drop-in centers where addicts can get counseling as well as material support for safe drug use, free from surveillance or intervention by law enforcement. Centers typically provide alcohol swabs, clean needles, and prep tins, which reduce risk of HIV and hepatitis among IV drug users; test strips for determining the purity of fentanyl and other drugs that are often adulterated by illicit drug dealers; and doses of Naloxone, a nasal spray that reduces the effects of opioids, and that has saved countless lives of persons who have overdosed. Dr. W points out that drop-in centers in some countries also provide medical supervision for persons who inject drugs on the premises, a practice that has recently been implemented at two centers in New York City.

When Dr. W concludes his remarks, he immediately sees that members of the council are skeptical. The council president, who is now in his fourth term, takes the lead, saying "I'm sorry doctor, but the last thing we need is to make it easier for people to use drugs. Many of our young people are rightly fearful of these drugs, and they also worry about getting caught breaking the law—providing them with a 'safe place' to do drugs sends the wrong message, and also undermines the efforts of law enforcement. All due respect, but this is not New York City." Other council members emphasize that their constituents would never tolerate a drop-in center in their neighborhoods, while deriding "big city, liberal solutions" to social problems.

Dr. W is disappointed in this response, but not really surprised. As he steps away from the podium, he says "This isn't about politics, council members, it's about saving lives and helping people in our community. I truly hope you will form a committee to study this idea before it is dismissed."

Questions

1. Do you agree with the claim that the proposed drop-in centers will encourage drug use and undermine law enforcement efforts?
2. Do you think the council should form a committee to study drop-in centers? If so, what factors should they consider in deciding whether to open a center in their community?
3. If you support drop-in centers that employ practical harm reduction strategies, what are the most serious concerns about such centers, and how would you address them? If you oppose such centers, what alternative would you support for treatment of patients with acute opioid use disorder?
4. Do differences between large urban settings as opposed to rural or small city settings affect whether drop-in centers should be adopted as one means of addressing the opioid crisis?

Resources

Goodnough, Abby. "Helping Drug Users Survive, Not Abstain: 'Harm Reduction' Gains Federal Support." *The New York Times,* June 27, 2021.

Mays, Jeffery C., and Andy Newman. "Nation's First Supervised Drug-Injection Sites Open in New York." *The New York Times*, November 30, 2021.

Nolen, Stephanie. "Fentanyl from the Government? A Vancouver Experiment Aims to Stop Overdoses." *The New York Times*, July 26, 2022.

Tyndall, Mark, and Zoë Dodd. "How Structural Violence, Prohibition, and Stigma Have Paralyzed North American Responses to Opioid Overdose." *AMA Journal of Ethics 22*, no. 8 (2020): E723–28. doi: 10.1001/amajethics.2020.723

7.12 Corporate Sponsorship of Public Health Initiatives

Keywords: conflict of interest

Dr. O is the medical commissioner of a department of health for one of the largest cities in the United States. In addition to providing sound medical guidance for the city's public health initiatives, Dr. O's job also involves navigating the complex web of relationships between public and private interests that make the city run. Although she is not an elected official, Dr. O realizes that her job is largely dependent on the goodwill of the city's mayor, who appoints the commissioner.

Dr. O has held the position of commissioner for just under two years now, but has served in a number of roles in the department over the last four years. In her time with the department, she has reinvigorated the department's work on public health equity in the city. One of her major projects has included a program that increases focus on mental health care for those in the justice system and provides services to those transitioning out of incarceration to help decrease recidivism. Although dedication of public resources to incarcerated people has not always been her most popular initiative politically, the mayor has largely supported it.

Every year, the department co-organizes the biggest public health event in the state. It is a summit that brings together public health experts, medical professionals, and lay persons for days of talks, education initiatives, free medical screenings, and other events to promote public health and increase engagement with the community. Dr. O has been asked to be the keynote speaker at the event to talk about her work with and for incarcerated persons.

Corporate sponsorships of large events like these are unavoidable, and the summit has received funding from a number of corporate partners in the past, including health care foundations, technology companies, and government consulting firms. Although Dr. O has always been uneasy about the ways in which corporate funding impacts health agendas, she also knows that in order to continue to have the outreach the department does, she must be willing to accept some level of nonpublic funding. As all partnerships up until this point have not presented immediate conflicts of interest and have always been publicly declared, she has been able to keep her concerns mainly to herself.

A few months before the summit this year, however, the mayor mentions the possibility of a new corporate sponsor, a multinational soft drink and convenience food company who promises to bring millions of dollars in funding to the event and has even intimated they would sponsor other public health initiatives. Although the company approached the mayor, Dr. O has final say over the organizing of the event, including accepting sponsorships. Dr. O is well versed in concerns about what are being called the "commercial determinants of health" in the public health literature. It has long been recognized in public health that noncommunicable diseases like diabetes and heart disease account for much of the disease burden across the world, especially in developed countries, and that the prevalence of these diseases in communities is in large part determined by social and economic circumstances beyond the control of those who struggle with the diseases. Dr. O is also aware of an emergent field of research on the role that global for-profit corporations play in the spread of noncommunicable disease, and the corporate sponsor the mayor is suggesting is one of the corporations whose impact on patterns of global health is thought to be the greatest. Dr. O wonders about the impact on public trust if she chooses to accept the funding that is being offered, but also realizes that the mayor would not have brought this offer to her if the mayor did not want it accepted.

Questions

1. Should Dr. O accept corporate funding for the event? What factors should she weigh in making this decision?
2. Would your reasoning about this case change if it was not an event being funded, but instead vaccinations for impoverished school children?

3. Under what circumstances, if any, do you think health officials should refuse corporate funding to support public health initiatives and events?

4. As governmental funding for health and public health research around the world has lessened, corporate funding for research has increased. What ethical issues might be involved in corporate sponsorship of scientific research?

Resources

Freudenberg, Nicholas. "Defining Appropriate Roles for Corporations in Public Health Research and Practice." *American Journal of Public Health* 108, no. 11 (2018): 1440–41. https://doi.org/10.2105/AJPH.2018.304714.

Lee, Kelley, and Nicholas Freudenberg. "Addressing the Commercial Determinants of Health Begins with Clearer Definition and Measurement." *Global Health Promotion* 27, no. 2 (2020): 3–5. https://doi.org/10.1177/1757975920931249.

Sorrel, Charlie. "Here Are All 96 Public Health Organizations Paid by Coca-Cola And Pepsi." *Fast Company*, October 13, 2016.

7.13 The Ethical Cost of Free Vaccines

Keywords: vaccines

In October 2016, the organization Doctors Without Borders turned down a donation from Pfizer of one million doses of PCV13, marketed as Prevnar 13. This vaccine inoculates against a normally fatal pneumonia. Worldwide, 1.4 million children a year die from this disease.

Prevnar 13 has been available since 2009. Pfizer has copyrights on the vaccine, as well as several on the processes used to produce the vaccine. Currently, only two companies manufacture the vaccine, Pfizer and GlaxoSmithKline (GSK). Doctors Without Borders has been interested in the vaccine since its release, but the price of the vaccine has always been too high to acquire the vaccine without donation.

The decision to turn down the vaccine did not come easy, according to Jason Cone, the Executive Director of Doctors Without Borders in the United States. While the donated vaccines would be useful, pharmaceutical companies often use donations to some organizations as justification for why prices remain high for others, including other humanitarian organizations and developing countries. These donations also often come with restrictions on the use of the vaccines. Moreover, the continued donation of vaccines crucial to the ongoing success of governmental and nongovernmental vaccination programs depends entirely on companies offering donations.

Instead of free Prevnar 13, Doctors Without Borders wants Pfizer to reduce the price of the vaccine so that they may purchase the vaccine when it is needed. A similar request and months of petitioning led GSK to lower the cost of the three-shot series to less than $10 for humanitarian organizations. While Pfizer has publicly committed to give up to 740 million of the vaccines at a discounted rate to Global Alliance for Vaccines and Immunization (GAVI) through 2025, it has refused to offer lower pricing to NGOs.

This might make good business sense, however, and this business sense might ultimately be a boon for vaccine production and creation. Vaccine development is expensive and historically the profit margin on vaccines has been quite low. Several decades ago, many pharmaceutical companies abandoned their vaccine divisions because there was not much profit to be made and many were losing money. The increase in the cost of vaccines over the past few years have brought an increase of profits for pharmaceutical companies, but it has also brought with it more investment in vaccine development. Moreover, even though profits have gone up, vaccine sales still only account for 2–3 percent of pharmaceutical company profits. Some economists argue that even with vaccines produced by pharmaceutical companies who have managed to make vaccine production profitable, lower prices on these vaccines have caused shortages in the U.S. market.

Questions

1. Was Doctors Without Borders justified in refusing the donation of these vaccines?
2. Do pharmaceutical companies have an obligation to provide vaccines and other lifesaving products to the developing world at a reduced cost? If so, what steps, if any, should be taken to encourage them to meet this obligation?
3. Corporations typically set prices for their products based on what a consumer will pay for that product. Is this practice appropriate for pharmaceuticals? If so, why? If not, what should be done to ensure that drugs are accessible to those who need them?

Resources

Cone, Jason. "There Is No Such Thing as 'Free' Vaccines: Why We Rejected Pfizer's Donation Offer of Pneumonia Vaccines." MSF Access Campaign-Medicines Are Not a Luxury (blog), October 10, 2016. https://msf-access.medium.com/there-is-no-such-thing-as-free-vaccines-why-we-rejected-pfizers-donation-offer-of-pneumonia-6a79c9d9f32f.

Emanuel, Ezekiel J. "When Is the Price of a Drug Unjust? The Average Lifetime Earnings Standard." *Health Affairs* 38, no. 4 (2019): 604–12. https://doi.org/10.1377/hlthaff.2018.05052.

Moodley, Keymanthri. "Vaccine Inequity Is Unethical." *Nature Human Behaviour* 6, no. 2 (2022): 168–69. https://doi.org/10.1038/s41562-022-01295-w.

Keyword Index

Abortion: 3.1, 3.2, 3.3, 3.4, 3.5, 3.6, 3.9

Addiction: 2.7, 5.5, 6.7, 6.14, 6.16, 7.8, 7.11

Advance directive: 2.9, 2.10, 2.11, 2.12, 2.13, 2.14, 5.2, 5.10

Alternative medicine: 1.3, 1.4, 1.11

Artificial intelligence: 4.11

Autonomy: 1.1, 1.2, 1.3, 1.5, 1.6, 1.8, 3.17, 5.7, 5.9, 6.13, 7.1

Bias: 2.15, 4.11, 6.5, 6.6, 6.7, 6.8, 6.9, 6.17, 7.3

Cancer: 1.3, 1.4, 1.5, 1.11, 2.1, 2.6, 2.12, 2.15, 3.11, 4.3

Capacity: 1.2, 2.2, 2.11, 2.12, 3.4, 5.3, 5.4, 5.9

Cardiopulmonary resuscitation: 2.3, 2.4, 7.4

Code status: 2.4, 5.10, 7.4

Coercion: 3.7, 3.10, 4.3, 4.4, 4.10, 5.9

Confidentiality: 1.20, 1.21, 3.8, 6.12, 7.8

Conflict of interest: 1.9, 1.10, 7.12

Consent: 1.11, 1.12, 1.13, 2.1, 2,2, 2.12, 3.4, 3.18, 4.1, 4.2, 4.3, 4.4, 4.7, 4.9, 4.10, 4.11, 4.12, 5.3, 5.6, 5,7, 6.16

Cost of care: 3.1, 3.3, 4.6, 6.1, 6.2, 6.3, 6.4

COVID-19: 2.14, 7.1, 7.3, 7.4, 7.5

Cultural difference: 1.13

Depression: 1.2, 1.3, 4.9, 5.2, 5.13

Difficult family: 1.19, 2.3

Difficult patient: 1.17, 1.18, 5.9

Disability: 1.19, 2.19, 3.4, 3.5, 3.13, 3.18

Duty to treat: 1.18

Duty to warn: 1.20, 5.12

End-of-life discussions: 2.1, 2.3, 2.4, 2.9, 2.16, 2.17

Eugenics: 3.10, 3.13, 3.14, 4.8

Futility: 2.3, 2.16, 2.17, 7.4

Gene editing: 4.8

Genetic testing: 1.21, 3.5, 3.6, 3.10, 3.12, 3.13, 3.14, 4.7

Health insurance: 4.6, 6.1, 6.3, 6.4

Heart disease: 1.16, 2.2, 2.3, 2.4, 2.8, 2.9, 2.11, 2.14, 6.6

Homelessness: 2.15, 5.4, 6.5

Human subject research: 4.1, 4.2, 4.3, 4.4, 4.5

Impaired infants: 2.18, 2.19, 2.20, 3.5, 3.6

In Vitro Fertilization: 3.11, 3.12, 3.13, 3.16

LGBTQ+ issues: 5.13, 6.13

Liability: 4.6, 4.11, 5.4

Maternal health: 3.2, 3.3, 3.5

Mental illness: 1.20, 2.11, 3.4, 5.1, 5.2, 5.8, 5.9, 5.10, 5.11, 5.12, 5.13, 6.4

Minors: 1.4, 1.5, 4.3, 4.5, 4.6, 6.13, 6.15

Moral distress: 2.4, 2.11, 2.19

Negligence: 1.15, 1.20

Nonadherence: 1.18, 5.1, 5.4, 5.8, 6.6, 7.8

Neurodegenerative disorder: 2.5, 2.13, 4.9, 4.12, 5.7

Nursing: 1.11, 1.12, 1.14, 1.15, 1.16, 1.17, 2.1, 5.5, 7.5

Obesity: 6.8, 6.9

Pain treatment: 5.5, 6.10

Palliative care: 2.6, 2.17

Parental authority: 1.4, 1.5, 1.7, 2.18, 2.19, 2.20, 4.6, 6.13, 6.15. 7.1

Paternalism: 1.1, 1.6, 1.8, 1.13, 3.16, 3.17, 3.18

Pediatrics: 1.4, 1.7, 2.18, 2.19, 2.20, 3.11, 7.1

Persistent vegetative state: 2.16,

Physician-assisted dying: 2.5, 2.6, 2.7, 2.8

Prenatal screening: 3.11, 3.12, 3.13, 3.14

Prescribing: 1.6, 1.7, 1.8, 1.9

Prisoners: 2.14, 4.1, 4.2, 6.16

Privacy: 1.21, 4.10, 4.12, 5.8, 6.16, 7.6, 7.8

Quarantine: 7.8, 7.9

Race: 1.17, 6.6, 6.10, 6.17, 7.3, 7.10

Refusal of care: 1.2, 1.3, 1.4, 1.5, 2.2

Religion: 2.3, 2.18, 3.5, 3.6, 5.3, 6.15

Resource allocation: 2.17, 5.1, 5.11, 6.7, 6.11, 7.3, 7.10

Rural health care: 2.5, 6.11, 6.12

Social determinants of health: 6.2, 6.3, 6.5, 6.14, 7.3, 7.10